"*Wonder Drug* is a delightful, informative story about the first round of psychedelic drug development. Carefully researched and beautifully presented, it concisely captures the history of this seminal period in a way that will bring a smile to any reader."

James W. Spisak, executive director of the Aldous and Laura Huxley Literary Trust

"*Wonder Drug* represents a glimpse into the pioneering research of psychedelic therapy, and those who paved the way for the new generation who are now picking up the torch. My own journey with psychedelic-assisted therapy would never have been possible without historians who kept the knowledge alive, and I greatly appreciate their efforts in not allowing the positive aspects of this treatment to be lost. If you don't know about Canada's groundbreaking work in the field of psychedelic-assisted therapy, then this is a great opportunity to expand your horizons and appreciate the efforts of these pioneers. One day, their work may help you or someone you care about."

Thomas Hartle, one of Canada's first legal users of psilocybin

"*Wonder Drug* is an important and fascinating tale charting the twentieth century rise of LSD research—with the help of North America's first socialist government—as a possible aid in combating schizophrenia, depression, and alcoholism. nicole marie burton's artwork is particularly stunning when depicting the psychedelic experiences of research volunteers."

David Lester, artist of the award-winning 1919: *A Graphic History of the Winnipeg General Strike*

"Brilliant! The history of psychedelics in graphic essay form. I had a great time reading it, learned many things I did not know, and greatly enjoyed the written section. It is at once entertaining and deep. This is a very useful contribution that brings together the many intertwining threads of the psychedelic era (up to today)."

Piero Ferrucci, psychotherapist and author

WONDER DRUG

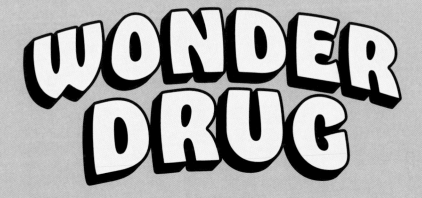

WONDER DRUG

LSD

in the Land
of Living Skies

Hugh D. A. Goldring
nicole marie burton

BASED ON THE RESEARCH OF DR. ERIKA DYCK

BETWEEN THE LINES

TORONTO

Wonder Drug
© 2021 Hugh D. A. Goldring and nicole marie burton

First published in 2021 by
Between the Lines
401 Richmond Street West, Studio 281
Toronto, Ontario, M5V 3A8, Canada
1-800-718-7201 · www.btlbooks.com

Library and Archives Canada Cataloguing in Publication

Title: Wonder drug : LSD in the land of living skies / written by Hugh D. A. Goldring ; illustrated by nicole marie burton ; based on the research of Dr. Erika Dyck.
Names: Goldring, Hugh, author. | Burton, Nicole Marie, artist.
Identifiers: Canadiana (print) 20210231726 | Canadiana (ebook) 20210231866 | ISBN 9781771135597 (softcover) | ISBN 9781771135603 (EPUB) | ISBN 9781771135610 (PDF)
Subjects: LCSH: Osmond, Humphry—Comic books, strips, etc. | LCSH: LSD (Drug)—Research—Saskatchewan—Weyburn—Comic books, strips, etc. | LCSH: Psychiatrists—Saskatchewan—Weyburn—Biography—Comic books, strips, etc. | LCGFT: Nonfiction comics. | LCGFT: Biographical comics.
Classification: LCC RC483.5.L9 G65 2021 | DDC 616.86/340270971244—dc23

Text and cover design by DEEVE
Printed in Canada

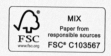

We acknowledge for their financial support of our publishing activities: the Government of Canada; the Canada Council for the Arts; and the Government of Ontario through the Ontario Arts Council, the Ontario Book Publishers Tax Credit program, and Ontario Creates.

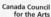

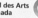

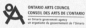
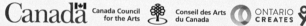

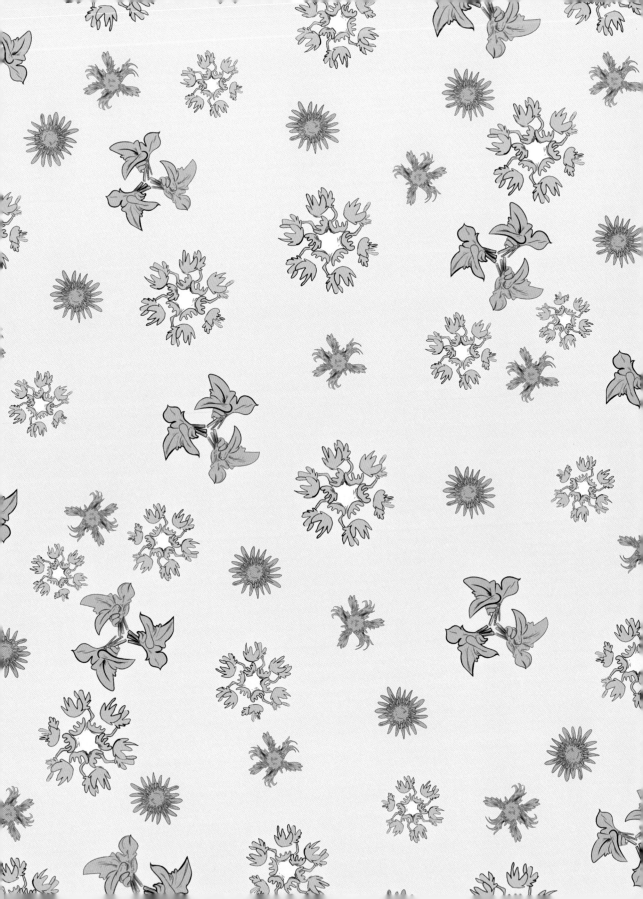

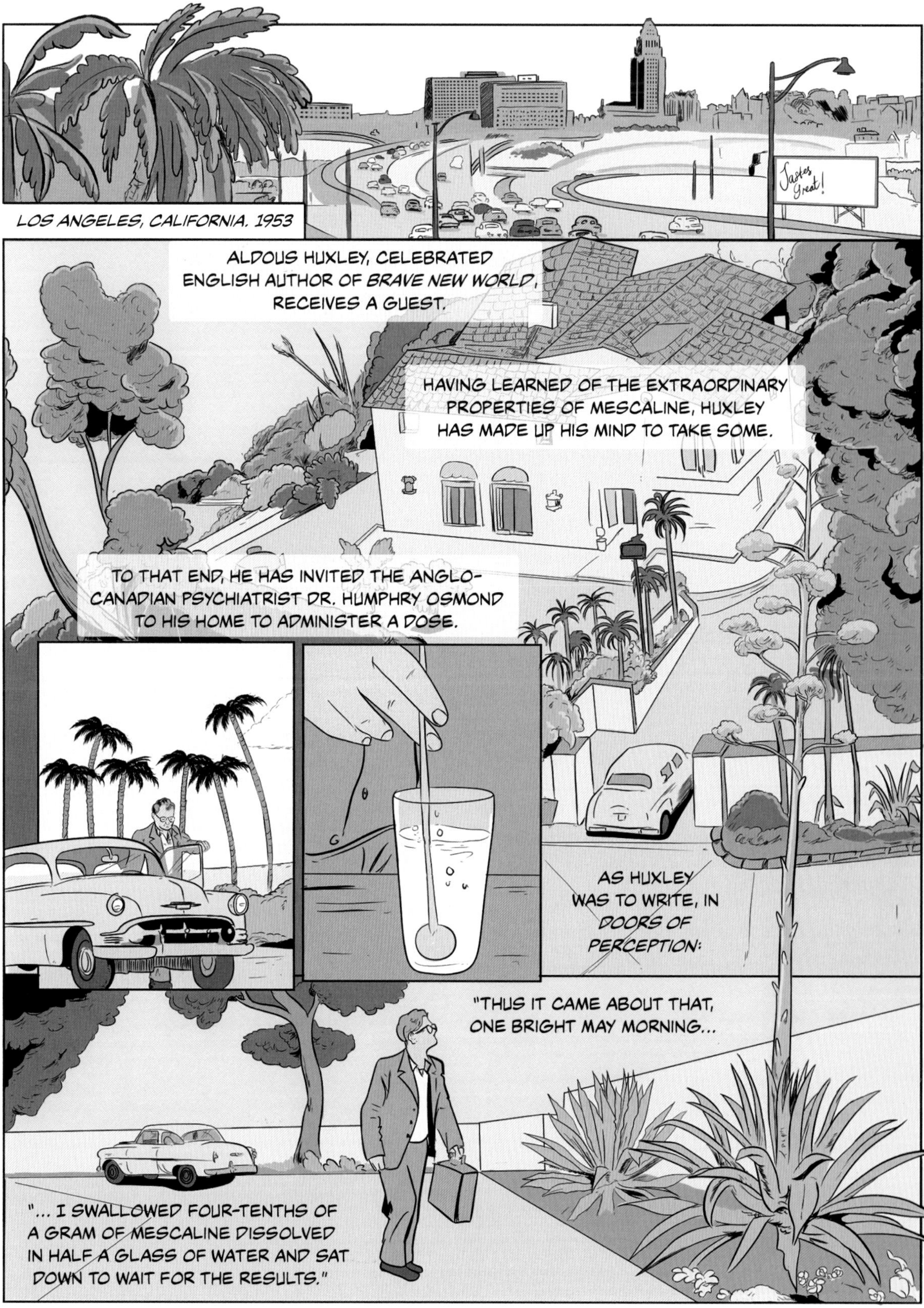

LOS ANGELES, CALIFORNIA, 1953
Tastes Great!
ALDOUS HUXLEY, CELEBRATED ENGLISH AUTHOR OF *BRAVE NEW WORLD*, RECEIVES A GUEST.
HAVING LEARNED OF THE EXTRAORDINARY PROPERTIES OF MESCALINE, HUXLEY HAS MADE UP HIS MIND TO TAKE SOME.
TO THAT END, HE HAS INVITED THE ANGLO-CANADIAN PSYCHIATRIST DR. HUMPHRY OSMOND TO HIS HOME TO ADMINISTER A DOSE.
AS HUXLEY WAS TO WRITE, IN *DOORS OF PERCEPTION*:
"THUS IT CAME ABOUT THAT, ONE BRIGHT MAY MORNING...
"... I SWALLOWED FOUR-TENTHS OF A GRAM OF MESCALINE DISSOLVED IN HALF A GLASS OF WATER AND SAT DOWN TO WAIT FOR THE RESULTS."

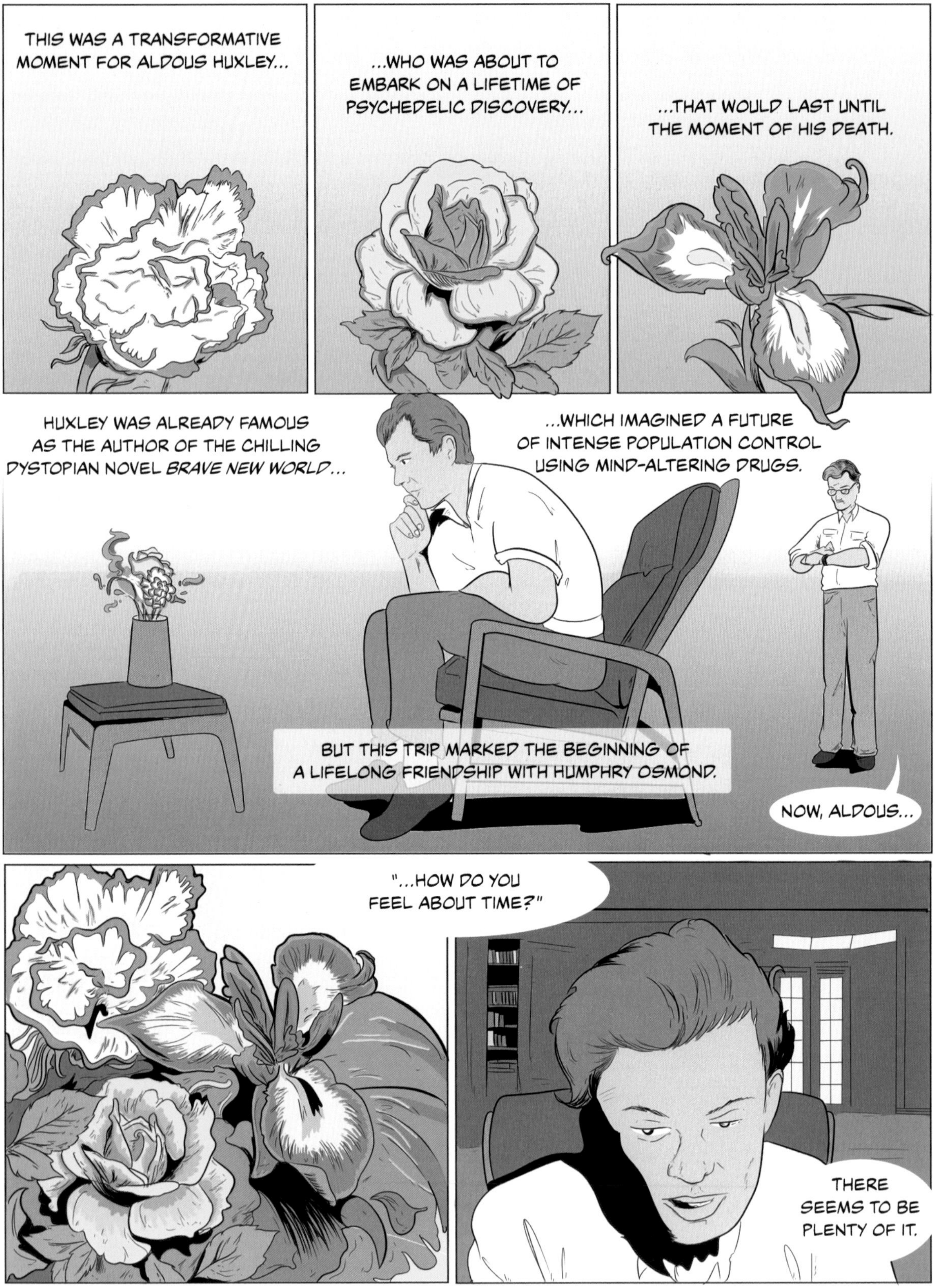
THIS WAS A TRANSFORMATIVE MOMENT FOR ALDOUS HUXLEY...
...WHO WAS ABOUT TO EMBARK ON A LIFETIME OF PSYCHEDELIC DISCOVERY...
...THAT WOULD LAST UNTIL THE MOMENT OF HIS DEATH.
HUXLEY WAS ALREADY FAMOUS AS THE AUTHOR OF THE CHILLING DYSTOPIAN NOVEL *BRAVE NEW WORLD*...
...WHICH IMAGINED A FUTURE OF INTENSE POPULATION CONTROL USING MIND-ALTERING DRUGS.
BUT THIS TRIP MARKED THE BEGINNING OF A LIFELONG FRIENDSHIP WITH HUMPHRY OSMOND.
NOW, ALDOUS...
"...HOW DO YOU FEEL ABOUT TIME?"
THERE SEEMS TO BE PLENTY OF IT.

IN FACT, THE TERM "PSYCHEDELIC" WAS COINED IN CORRESPONDENCE BETWEEN THE TWO.

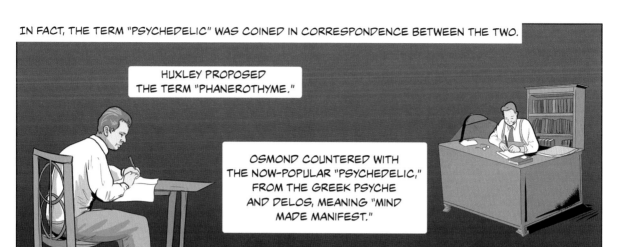

HUXLEY PROPOSED THE TERM "PHANEROTHYME."

OSMOND COUNTERED WITH THE NOW-POPULAR "PSYCHEDELIC," FROM THE GREEK PSYCHE AND DELOS, MEANING "MIND MADE MANIFEST."

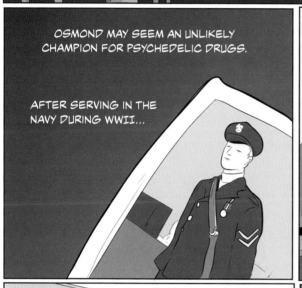

OSMOND MAY SEEM AN UNLIKELY CHAMPION FOR PSYCHEDELIC DRUGS.

AFTER SERVING IN THE NAVY DURING WWII...

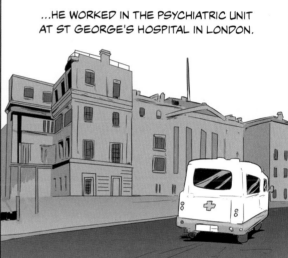

...HE WORKED IN THE PSYCHIATRIC UNIT AT ST GEORGE'S HOSPITAL IN LONDON.

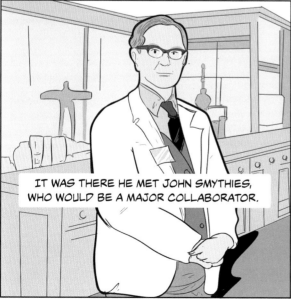

IT WAS THERE HE MET JOHN SMYTHIES, WHO WOULD BE A MAJOR COLLABORATOR.

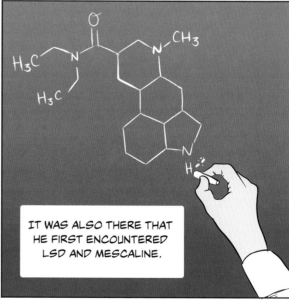

IT WAS ALSO THERE THAT HE FIRST ENCOUNTERED LSD AND MESCALINE.

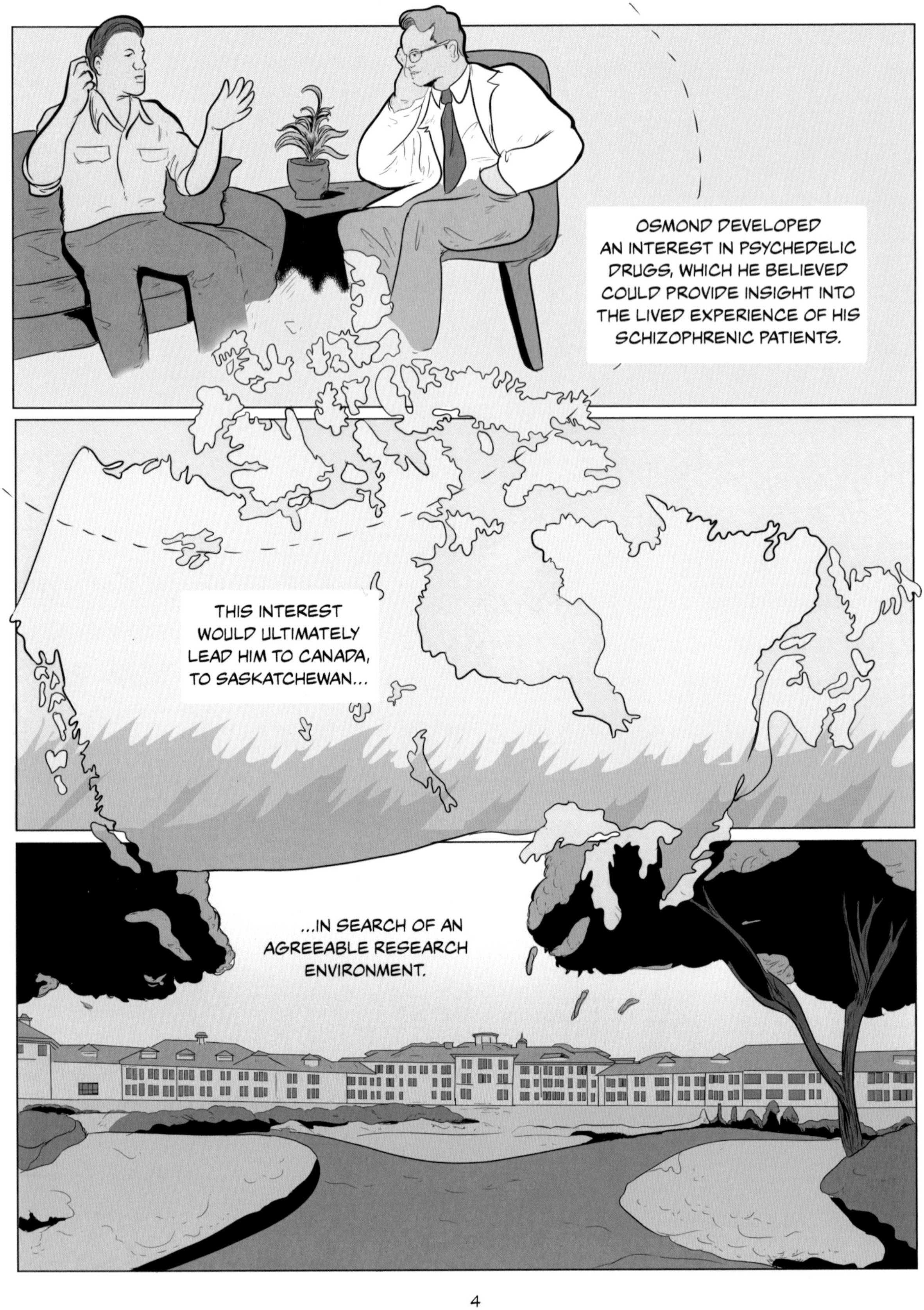
OSMOND DEVELOPED AN INTEREST IN PSYCHEDELIC DRUGS, WHICH HE BELIEVED COULD PROVIDE INSIGHT INTO THE LIVED EXPERIENCE OF HIS SCHIZOPHRENIC PATIENTS.
THIS INTEREST WOULD ULTIMATELY LEAD HIM TO CANADA, TO SASKATCHEWAN...
...IN SEARCH OF AN AGREEABLE RESEARCH ENVIRONMENT.

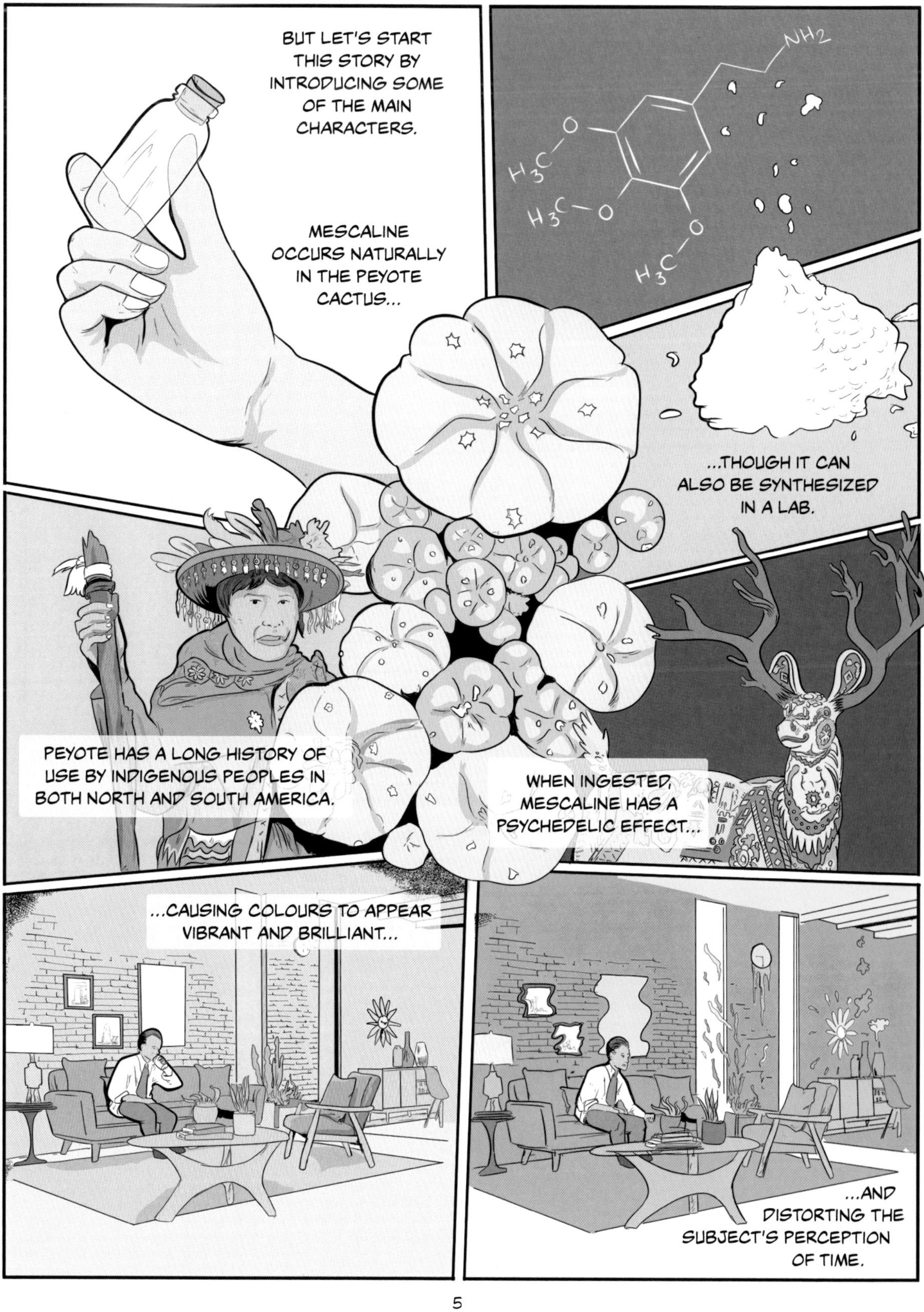
BUT LET'S START THIS STORY BY INTRODUCING SOME OF THE MAIN CHARACTERS.
MESCALINE OCCURS NATURALLY IN THE PEYOTE CACTUS...
NH2
H3C O
H3C O
H3C O
...THOUGH IT CAN ALSO BE SYNTHESIZED IN A LAB.
PEYOTE HAS A LONG HISTORY OF USE BY INDIGENOUS PEOPLES IN BOTH NORTH AND SOUTH AMERICA.
WHEN INGESTED, MESCALINE HAS A PSYCHEDELIC EFFECT...
...CAUSING COLOURS TO APPEAR VIBRANT AND BRILLIANT...
...AND DISTORTING THE SUBJECT'S PERCEPTION OF TIME.

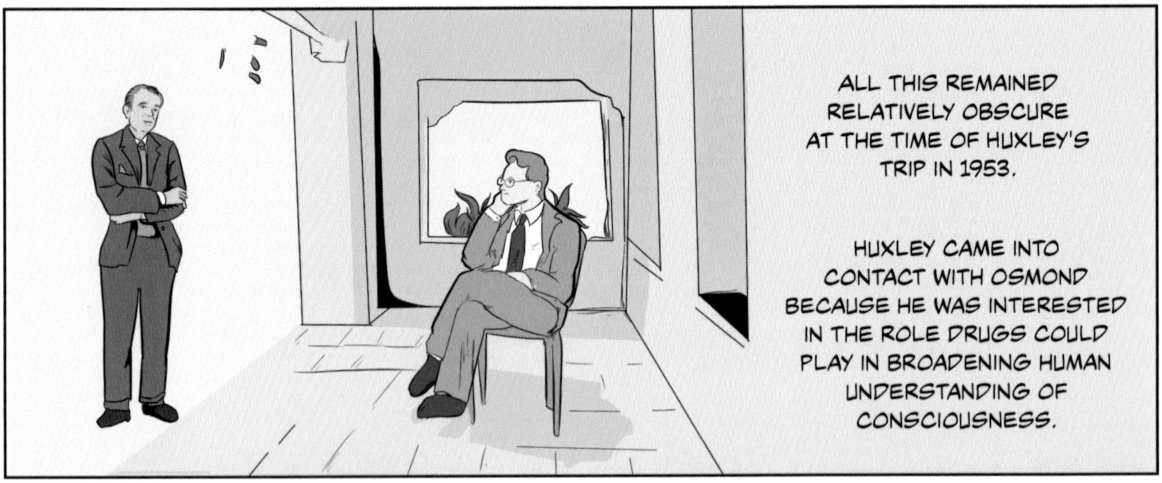
ALL THIS REMAINED RELATIVELY OBSCURE AT THE TIME OF HUXLEY'S TRIP IN 1953.
HUXLEY CAME INTO CONTACT WITH OSMOND BECAUSE HE WAS INTERESTED IN THE ROLE DRUGS COULD PLAY IN BROADENING HUMAN UNDERSTANDING OF CONSCIOUSNESS.

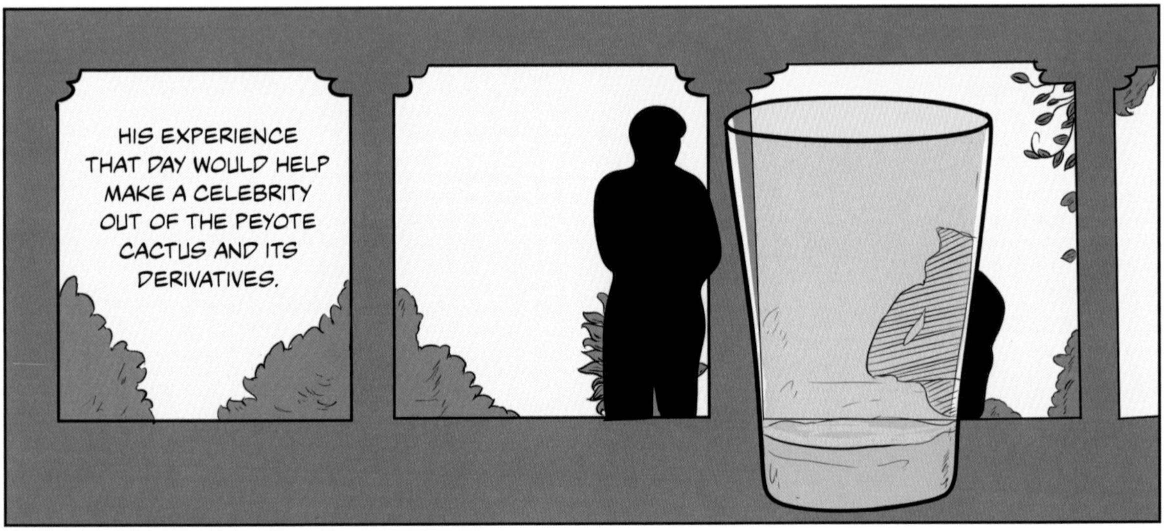
HIS EXPERIENCE THAT DAY WOULD HELP MAKE A CELEBRITY OUT OF THE PEYOTE CACTUS AND ITS DERIVATIVES.

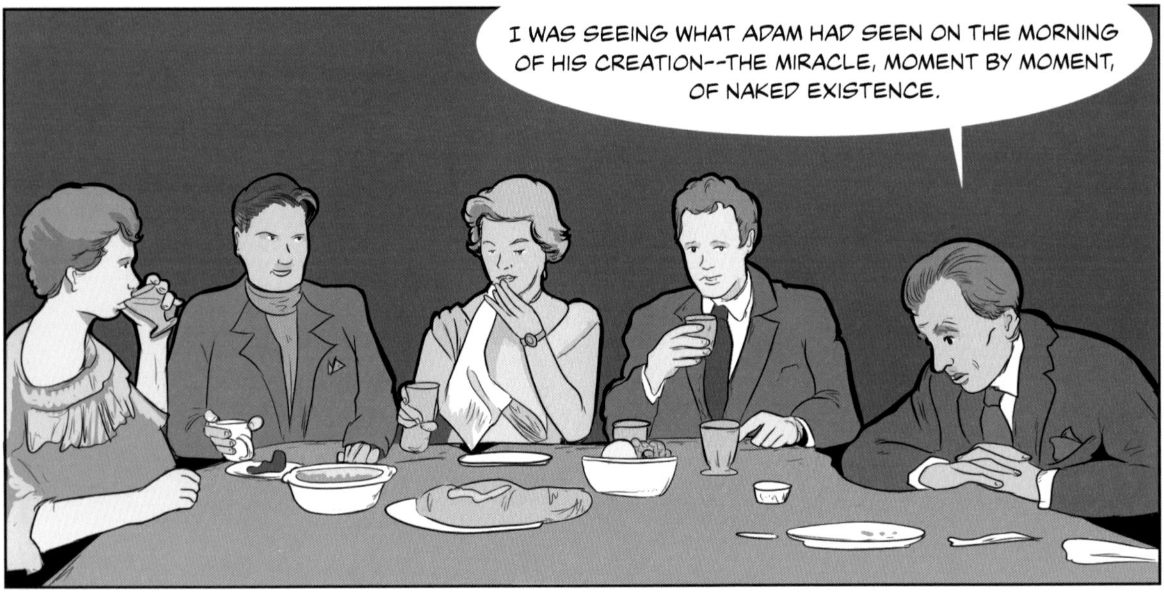
I WAS SEEING WHAT ADAM HAD SEEN ON THE MORNING OF HIS CREATION--THE MIRACLE, MOMENT BY MOMENT, OF NAKED EXISTENCE.

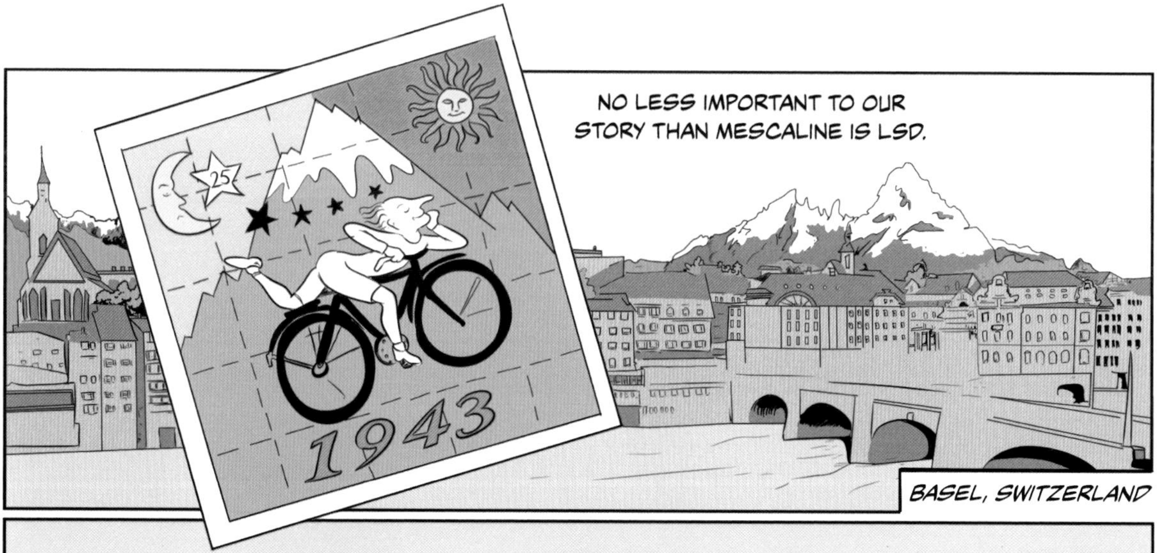

NO LESS IMPORTANT TO OUR STORY THAN MESCALINE IS LSD.
25
1943
BASEL, SWITZERLAND

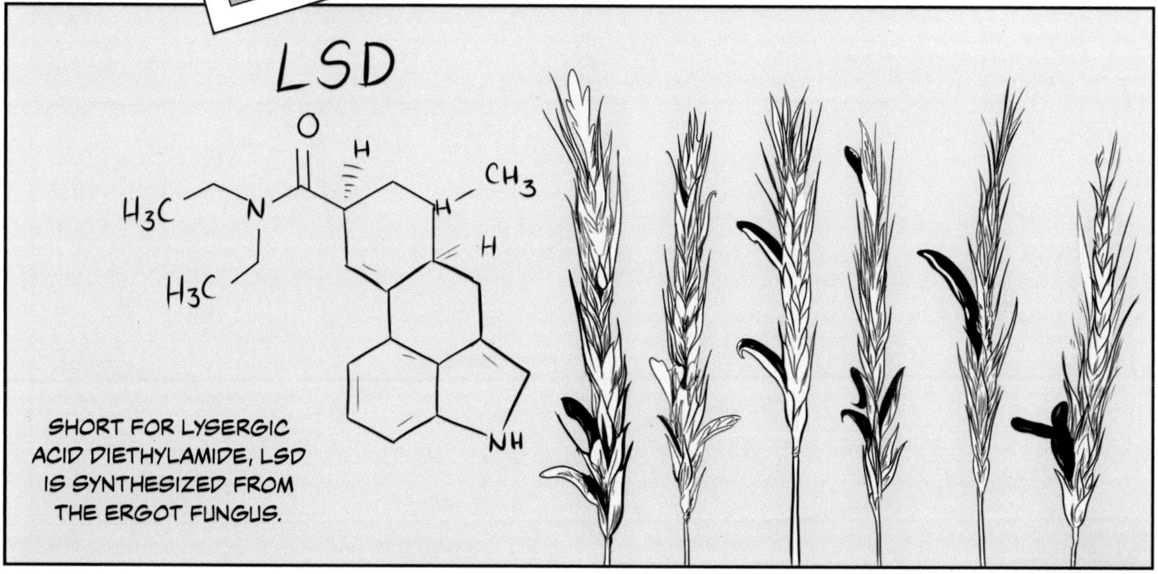

LSD
SHORT FOR LYSERGIC ACID DIETHYLAMIDE, LSD IS SYNTHESIZED FROM THE ERGOT FUNGUS.

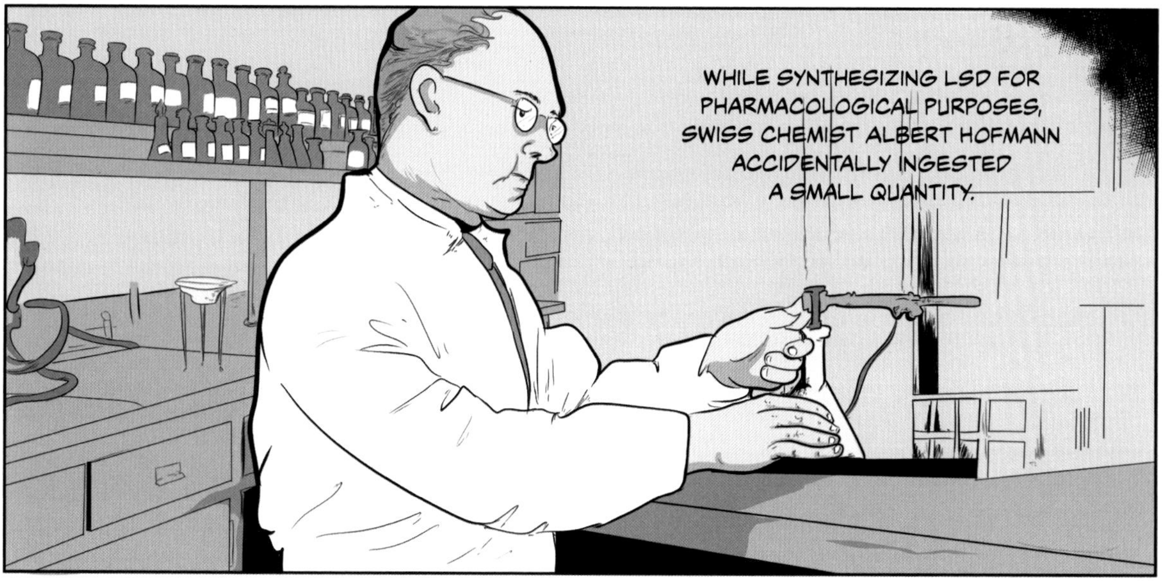

WHILE SYNTHESIZING LSD FOR PHARMACOLOGICAL PURPOSES, SWISS CHEMIST ALBERT HOFMANN ACCIDENTALLY INGESTED A SMALL QUANTITY.

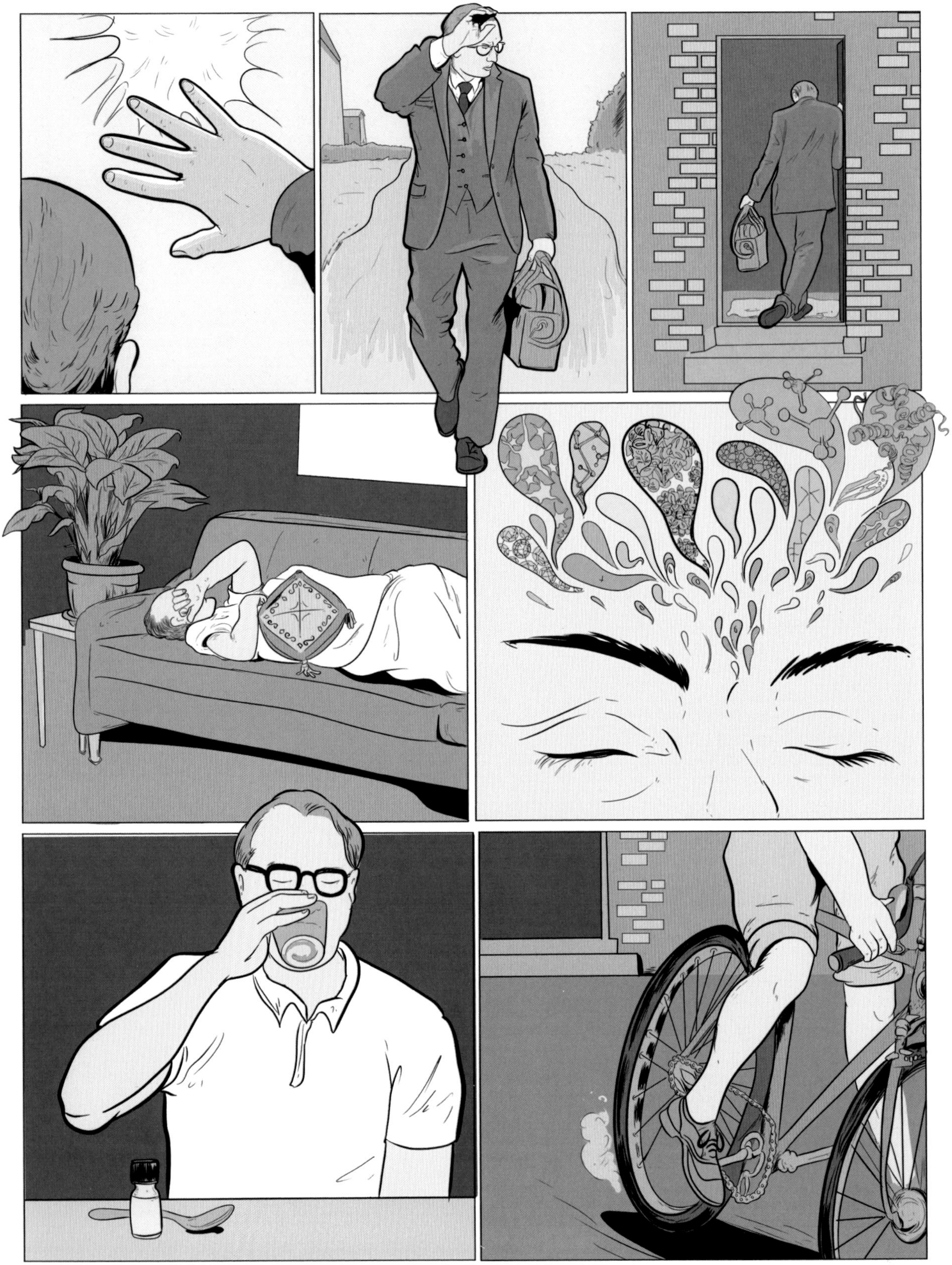

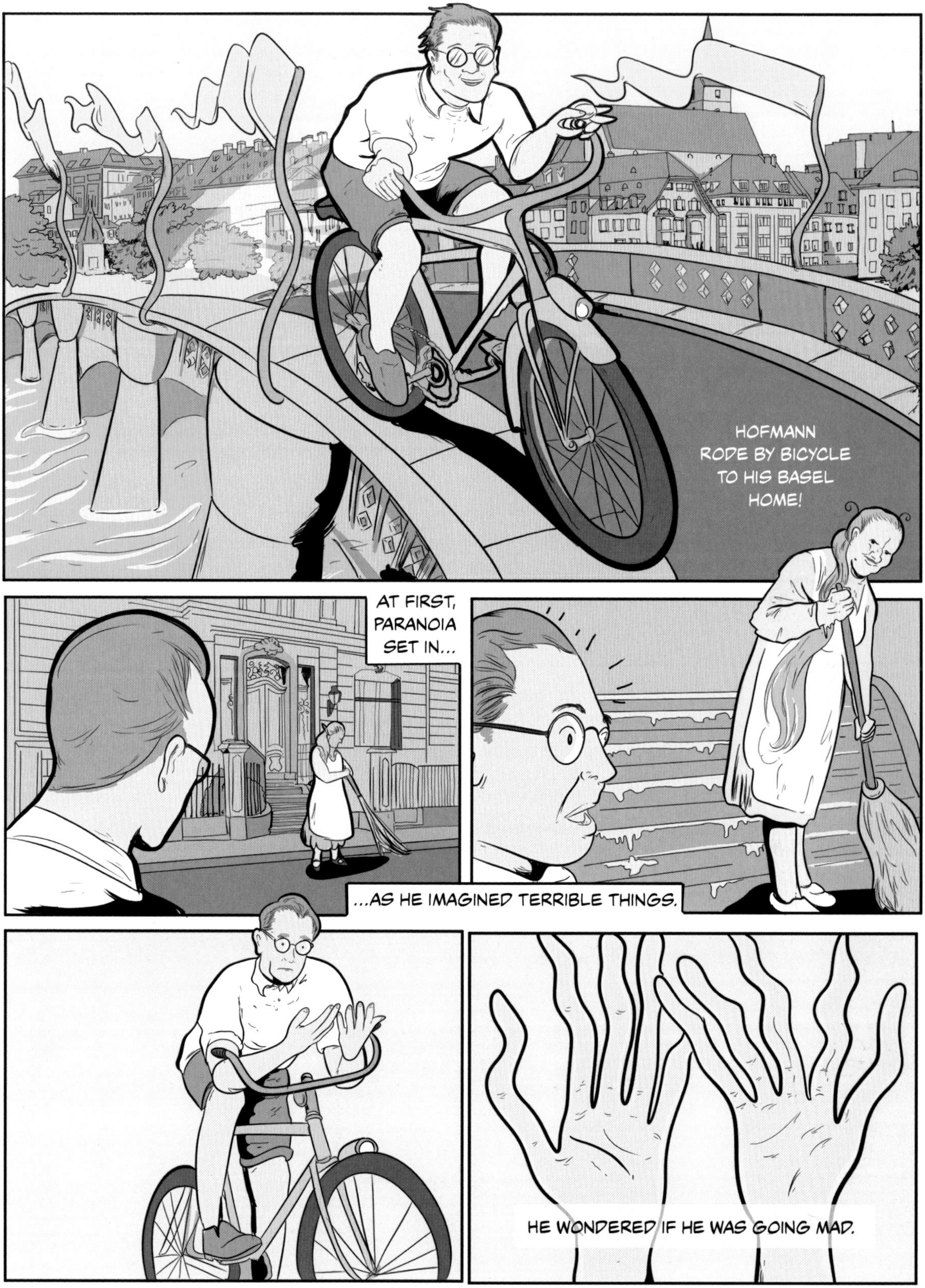
HOFMANN RODE BY BICYCLE TO HIS BASEL HOME!
AT FIRST, PARANOIA SET IN...
...AS HE IMAGINED TERRIBLE THINGS.
HE WONDERED IF HE WAS GOING MAD.

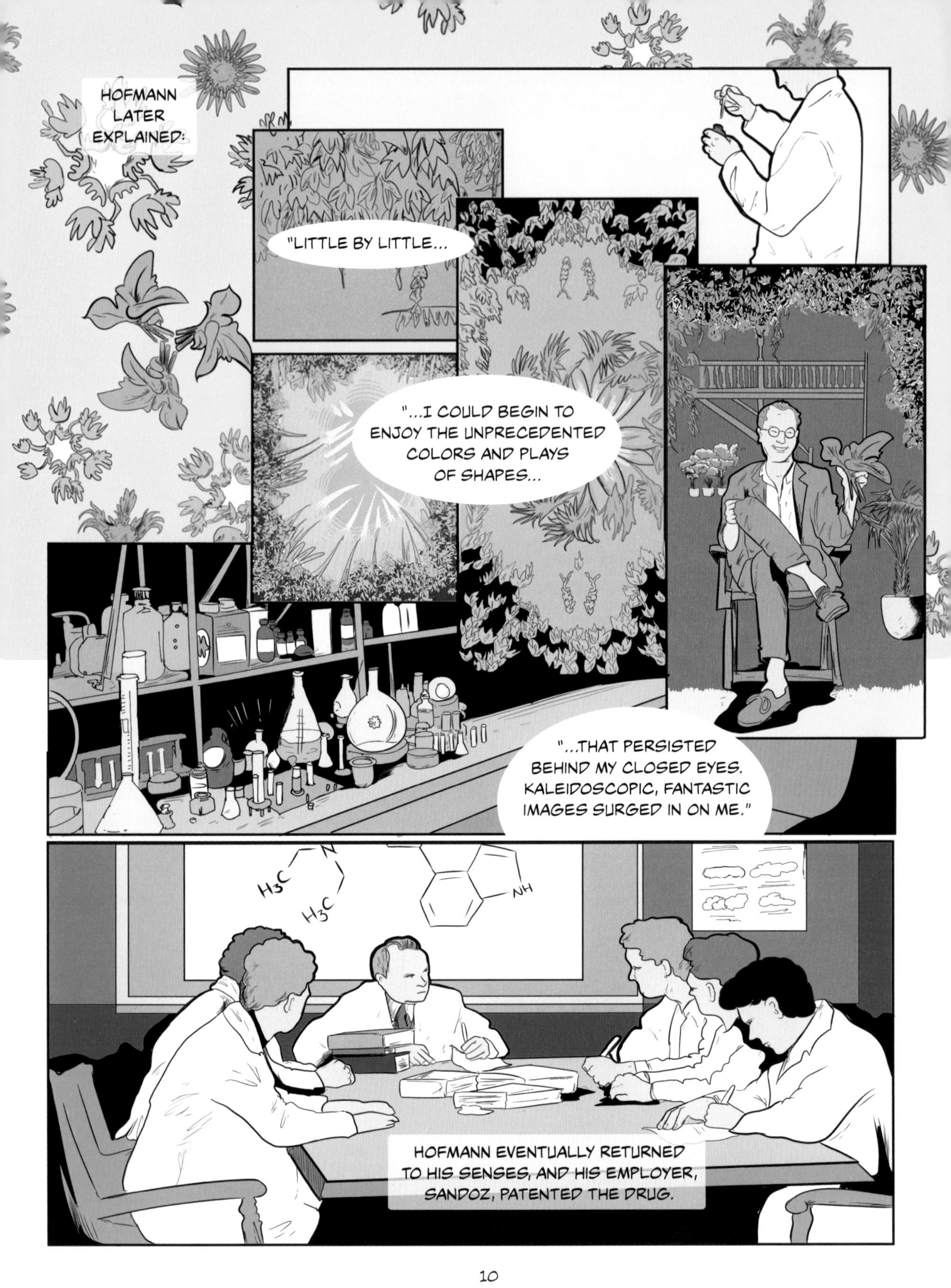

HOFMANN LATER EXPLAINED:
"LITTLE BY LITTLE...
"...I COULD BEGIN TO ENJOY THE UNPRECEDENTED COLORS AND PLAYS OF SHAPES...
"...THAT PERSISTED BEHIND MY CLOSED EYES. KALEIDOSCOPIC, FANTASTIC IMAGES SURGED IN ON ME."
H_3C
H_3C
NH
HOFMANN EVENTUALLY RETURNED TO HIS SENSES, AND HIS EMPLOYER, SANDOZ, PATENTED THE DRUG.

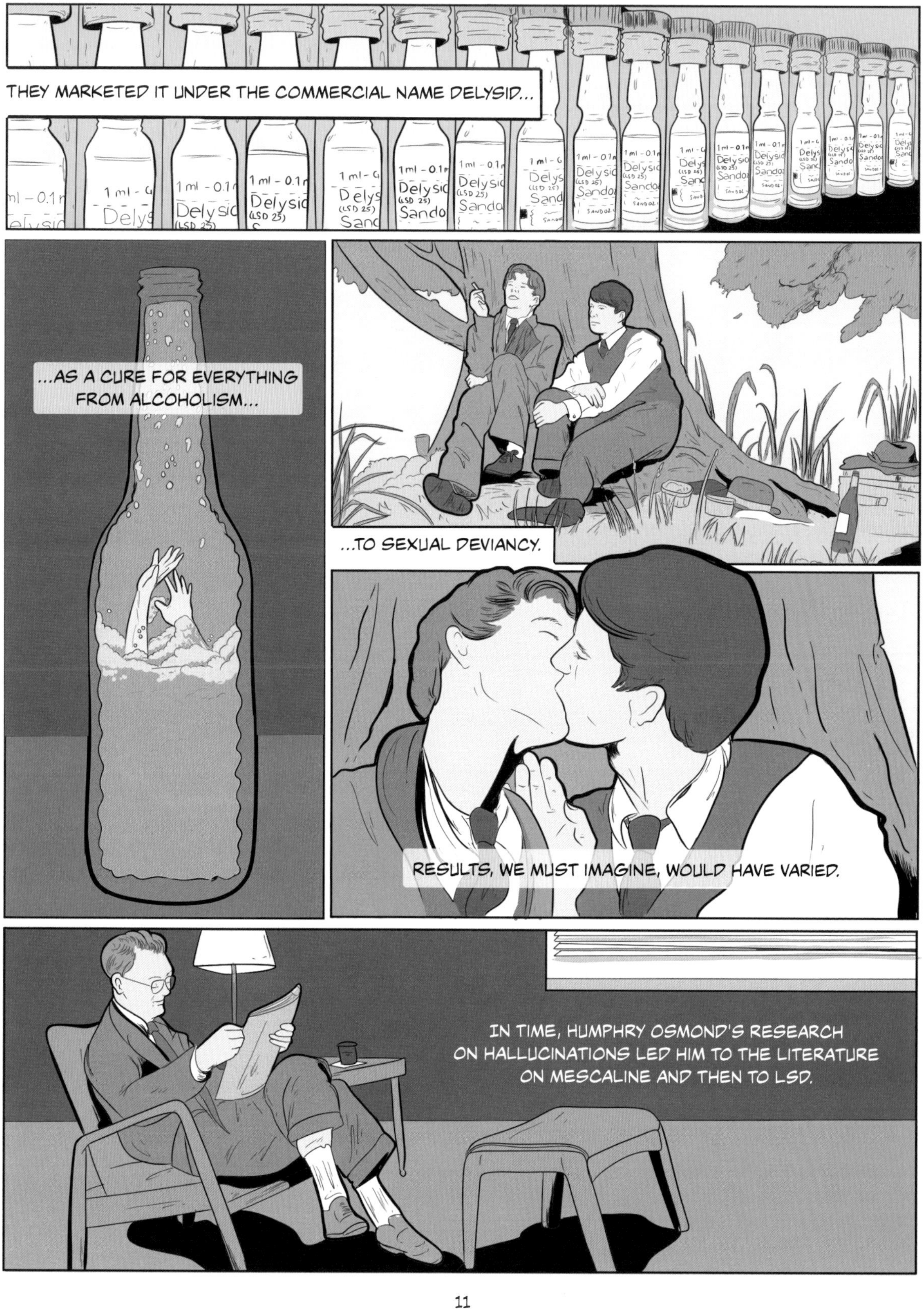
THEY MARKETED IT UNDER THE COMMERCIAL NAME DELYSID...
...AS A CURE FOR EVERYTHING FROM ALCOHOLISM...
...TO SEXUAL DEVIANCY.
RESULTS, WE MUST IMAGINE, WOULD HAVE VARIED.
IN TIME, HUMPHRY OSMOND'S RESEARCH ON HALLUCINATIONS LED HIM TO THE LITERATURE ON MESCALINE AND THEN TO LSD.

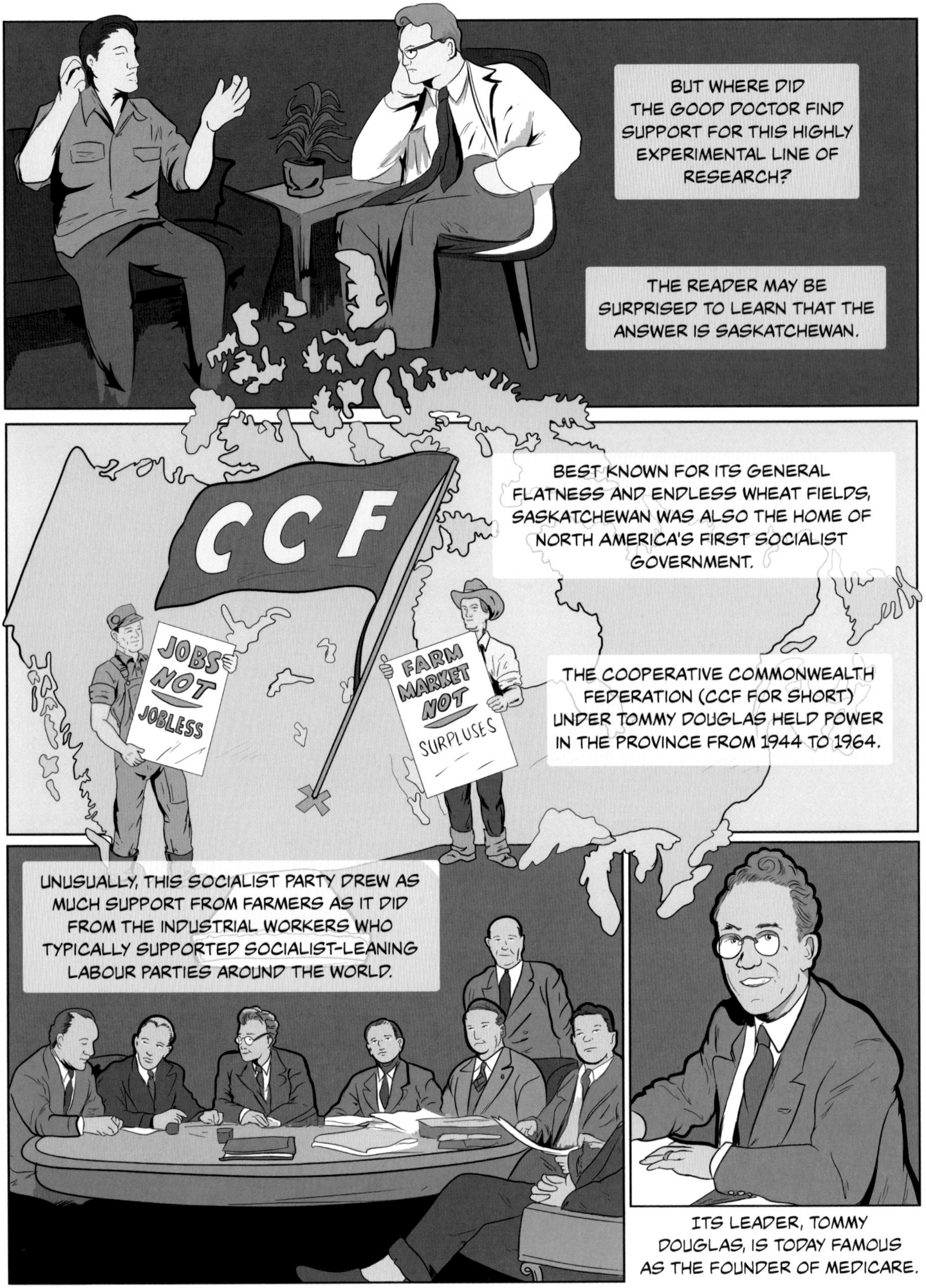
BUT WHERE DID THE GOOD DOCTOR FIND SUPPORT FOR THIS HIGHLY EXPERIMENTAL LINE OF RESEARCH?
THE READER MAY BE SURPRISED TO LEARN THAT THE ANSWER IS SASKATCHEWAN.
BEST KNOWN FOR ITS GENERAL FLATNESS AND ENDLESS WHEAT FIELDS, SASKATCHEWAN WAS ALSO THE HOME OF NORTH AMERICA'S FIRST SOCIALIST GOVERNMENT.
CCF
JOBS NOT JOBLESS
FARM MARKET NOT SURPLUSES
THE COOPERATIVE COMMONWEALTH FEDERATION (CCF FOR SHORT) UNDER TOMMY DOUGLAS HELD POWER IN THE PROVINCE FROM 1944 TO 1964.
UNUSUALLY, THIS SOCIALIST PARTY DREW AS MUCH SUPPORT FROM FARMERS AS IT DID FROM THE INDUSTRIAL WORKERS WHO TYPICALLY SUPPORTED SOCIALIST-LEANING LABOUR PARTIES AROUND THE WORLD.
ITS LEADER, TOMMY DOUGLAS, IS TODAY FAMOUS AS THE FOUNDER OF MEDICARE.

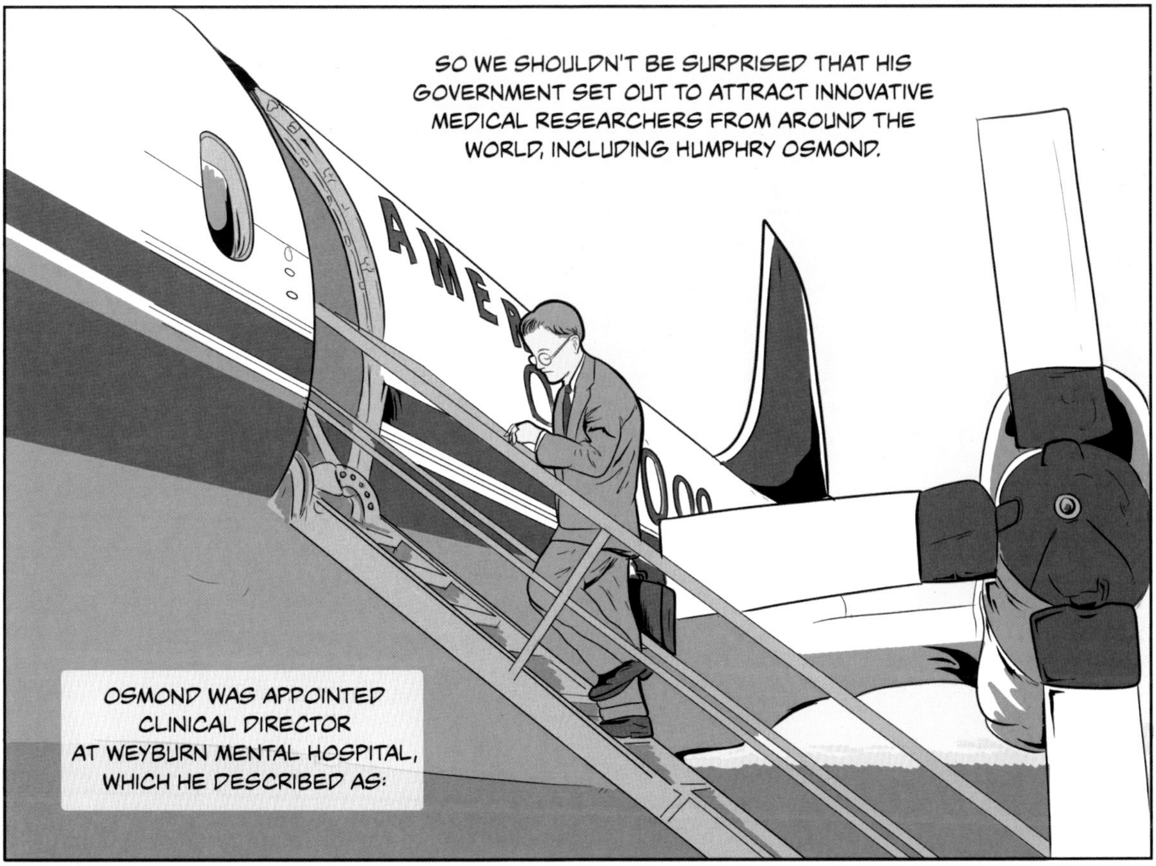
SO WE SHOULDN'T BE SURPRISED THAT HIS GOVERNMENT SET OUT TO ATTRACT INNOVATIVE MEDICAL RESEARCHERS FROM AROUND THE WORLD, INCLUDING HUMPHRY OSMOND.
OSMOND WAS APPOINTED CLINICAL DIRECTOR AT WEYBURN MENTAL HOSPITAL, WHICH HE DESCRIBED AS:

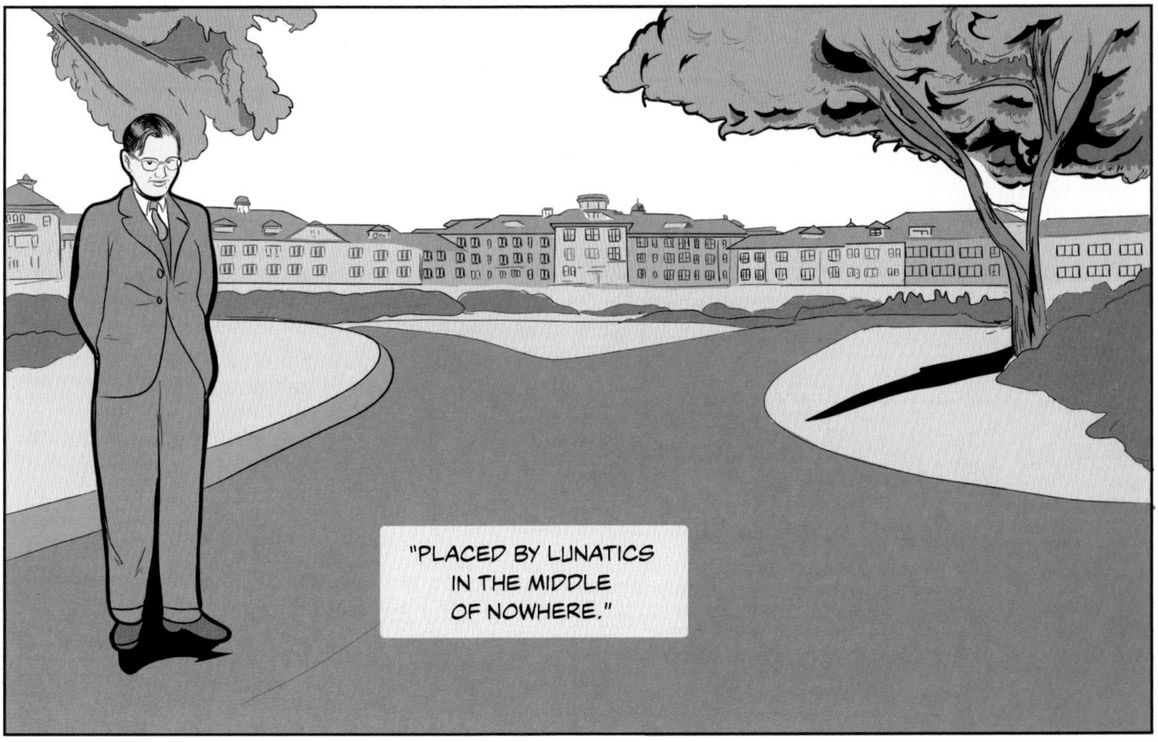
"PLACED BY LUNATICS IN THE MIDDLE OF NOWHERE."

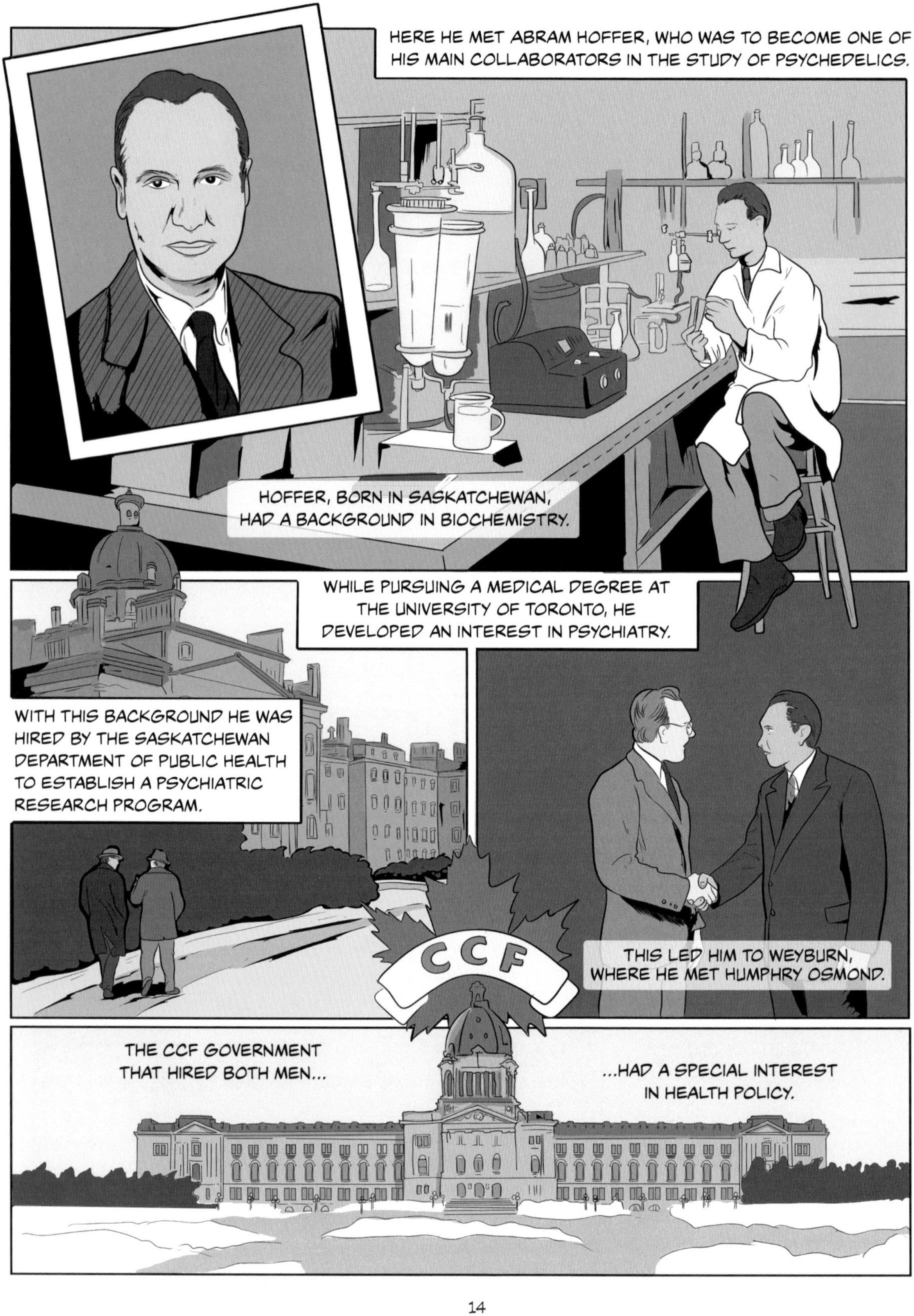
HERE HE MET ABRAM HOFFER, WHO WAS TO BECOME ONE OF HIS MAIN COLLABORATORS IN THE STUDY OF PSYCHEDELICS.
HOFFER, BORN IN SASKATCHEWAN, HAD A BACKGROUND IN BIOCHEMISTRY.
WHILE PURSUING A MEDICAL DEGREE AT THE UNIVERSITY OF TORONTO, HE DEVELOPED AN INTEREST IN PSYCHIATRY.
WITH THIS BACKGROUND HE WAS HIRED BY THE SASKATCHEWAN DEPARTMENT OF PUBLIC HEALTH TO ESTABLISH A PSYCHIATRIC RESEARCH PROGRAM.
CCF
THIS LED HIM TO WEYBURN, WHERE HE MET HUMPHRY OSMOND.
THE CCF GOVERNMENT THAT HIRED BOTH MEN...
...HAD A SPECIAL INTEREST IN HEALTH POLICY.

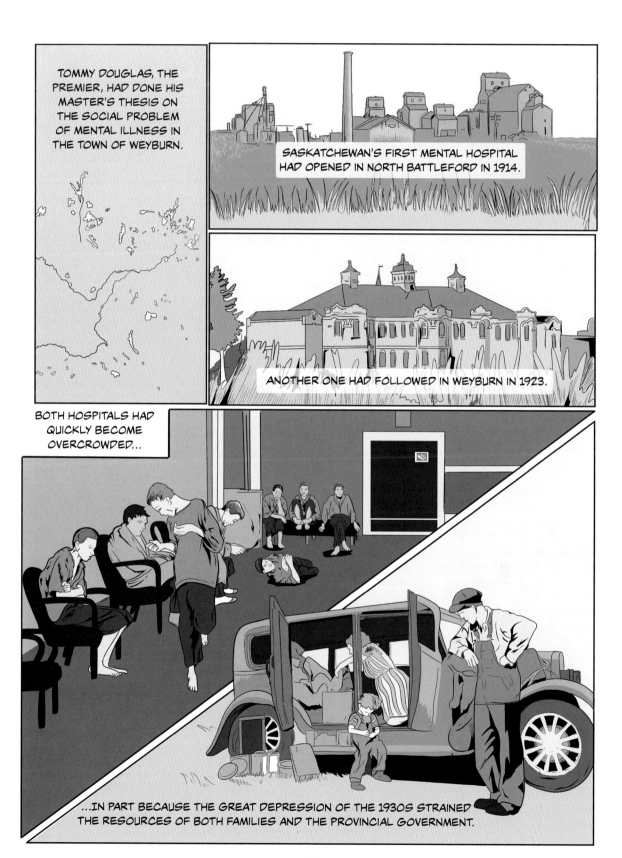

TOMMY DOUGLAS, THE PREMIER, HAD DONE HIS MASTER'S THESIS ON THE SOCIAL PROBLEM OF MENTAL ILLNESS IN THE TOWN OF WEYBURN.

SASKATCHEWAN'S FIRST MENTAL HOSPITAL HAD OPENED IN NORTH BATTLEFORD IN 1914.

ANOTHER ONE HAD FOLLOWED IN WEYBURN IN 1923.

BOTH HOSPITALS HAD QUICKLY BECOME OVERCROWDED...

...IN PART BECAUSE THE GREAT DEPRESSION OF THE 1930S STRAINED THE RESOURCES OF BOTH FAMILIES AND THE PROVINCIAL GOVERNMENT.

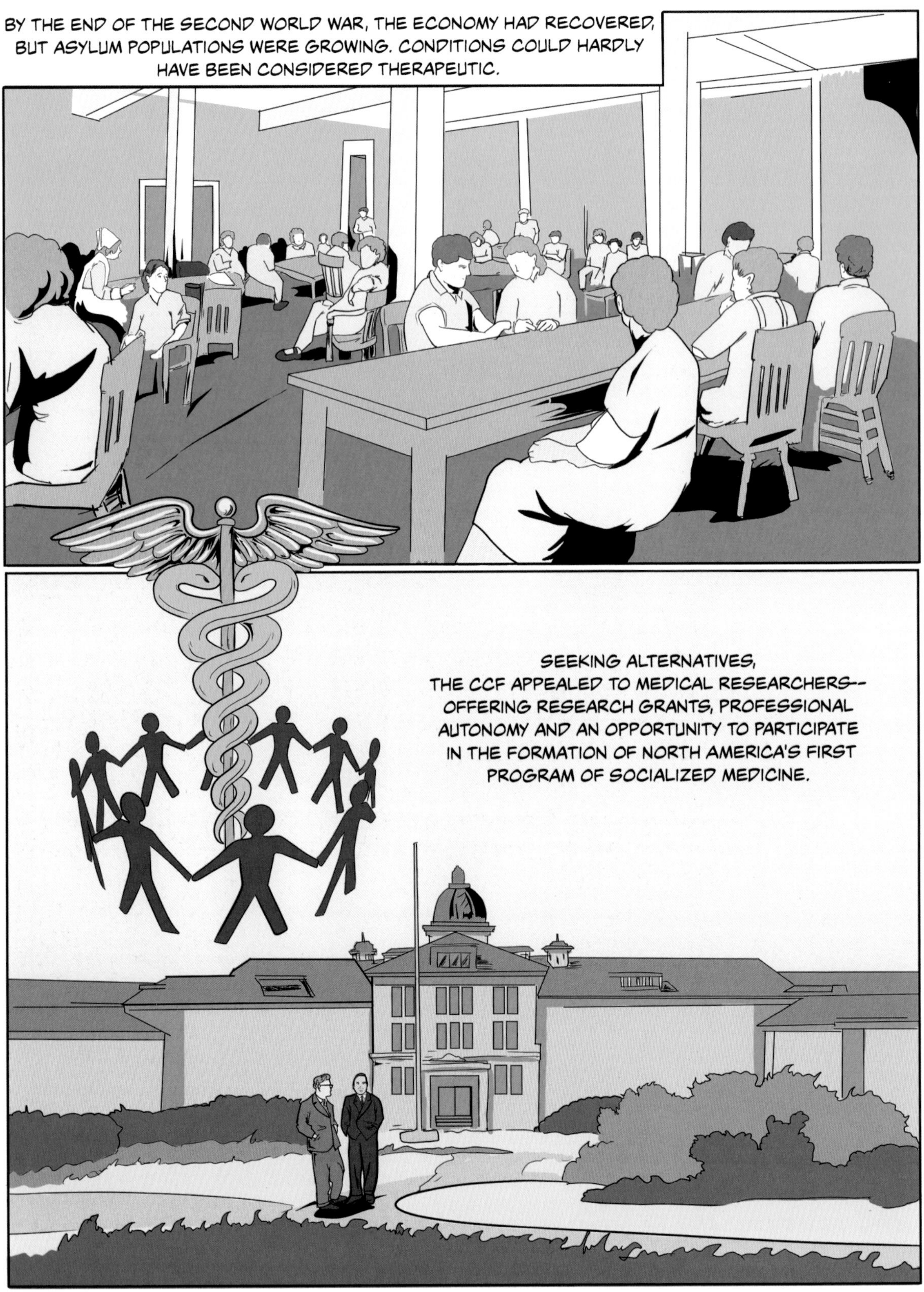
BY THE END OF THE SECOND WORLD WAR, THE ECONOMY HAD RECOVERED, BUT ASYLUM POPULATIONS WERE GROWING. CONDITIONS COULD HARDLY HAVE BEEN CONSIDERED THERAPEUTIC.
SEEKING ALTERNATIVES, THE CCF APPEALED TO MEDICAL RESEARCHERS-- OFFERING RESEARCH GRANTS, PROFESSIONAL AUTONOMY AND AN OPPORTUNITY TO PARTICIPATE IN THE FORMATION OF NORTH AMERICA'S FIRST PROGRAM OF SOCIALIZED MEDICINE.

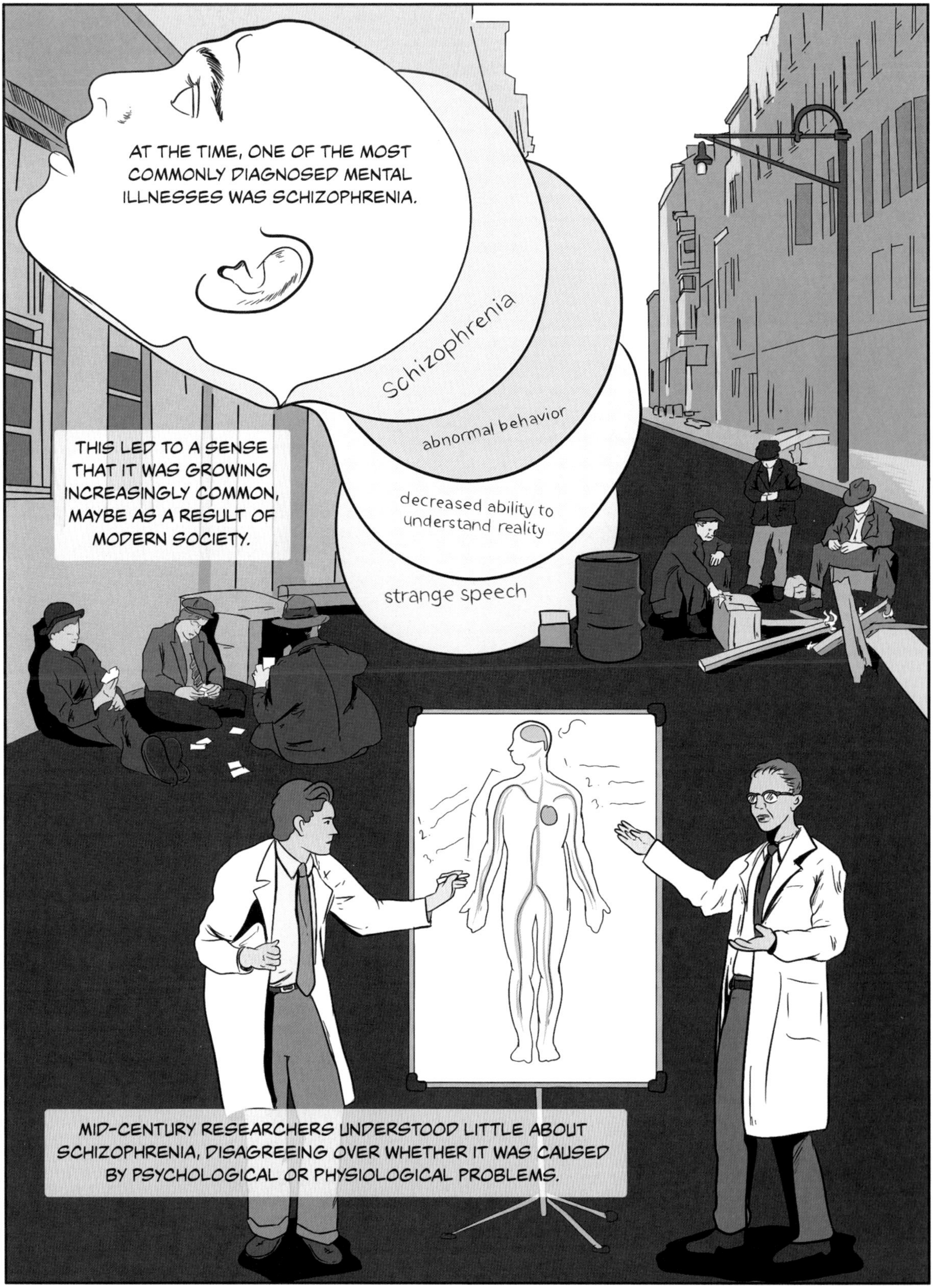

AT THE TIME, ONE OF THE MOST COMMONLY DIAGNOSED MENTAL ILLNESSES WAS SCHIZOPHRENIA.
schizophrenia
abnormal behavior
decreased ability to understand reality
strange speech
THIS LED TO A SENSE THAT IT WAS GROWING INCREASINGLY COMMON, MAYBE AS A RESULT OF MODERN SOCIETY.
MID-CENTURY RESEARCHERS UNDERSTOOD LITTLE ABOUT SCHIZOPHRENIA, DISAGREEING OVER WHETHER IT WAS CAUSED BY PSYCHOLOGICAL OR PHYSIOLOGICAL PROBLEMS.

ONE POPULAR TREATMENT WAS ELECTROCONVULSIVE THERAPY, WHICH INVOLVED ELECTRICALLY INDUCED SEIZURES IN THE PATIENT'S BRAIN.

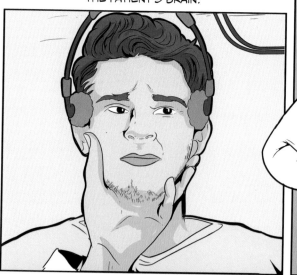

OSMOND WAS SKEPTICAL OF THE EFFECTIVENESS OF ECT.

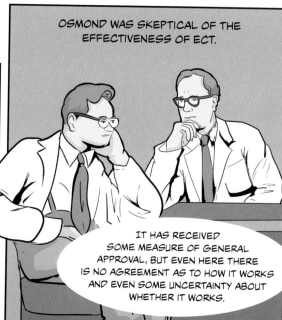

IT HAS RECEIVED SOME MEASURE OF GENERAL APPROVAL, BUT EVEN HERE THERE IS NO AGREEMENT AS TO HOW IT WORKS AND EVEN SOME UNCERTAINTY ABOUT WHETHER IT WORKS.

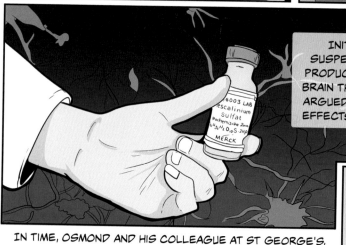

INITIALLY, OSMOND AND HOFFMAN SUSPECTED THAT A METABOLIC FAILURE PRODUCED AN UNKNOWN CHEMICAL IN THE BRAIN THAT CAUSED SCHIZOPHRENIA. THEY ARGUED THAT MESCALINE SIMULATED THE EFFECTS OF THIS THEORIZED SUBSTANCE.

IN TIME, OSMOND AND HIS COLLEAGUE AT ST GEORGE'S, JOHN SMYTHIES, DEVELOPED A HYBRID EXPLANATION...

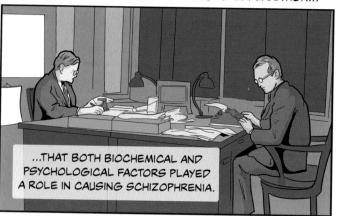

...THAT BOTH BIOCHEMICAL AND PSYCHOLOGICAL FACTORS PLAYED A ROLE IN CAUSING SCHIZOPHRENIA.

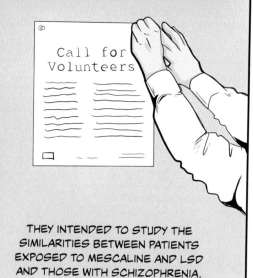

Call for Volunteers

THEY INTENDED TO STUDY THE SIMILARITIES BETWEEN PATIENTS EXPOSED TO MESCALINE AND LSD AND THOSE WITH SCHIZOPHRENIA.

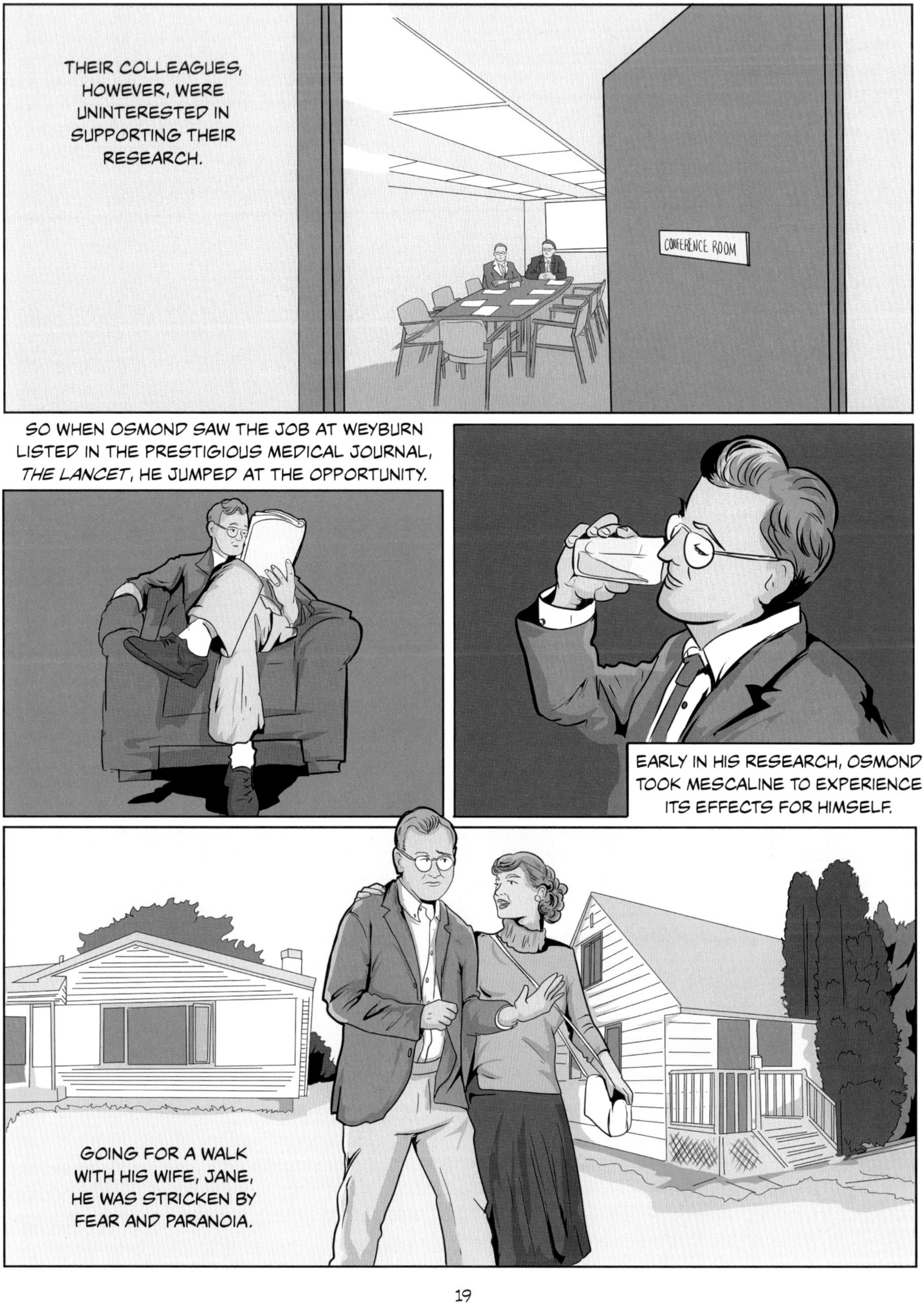
THEIR COLLEAGUES, HOWEVER, WERE UNINTERESTED IN SUPPORTING THEIR RESEARCH.
CONFERENCE ROOM
SO WHEN OSMOND SAW THE JOB AT WEYBURN LISTED IN THE PRESTIGIOUS MEDICAL JOURNAL, *THE LANCET*, HE JUMPED AT THE OPPORTUNITY.
EARLY IN HIS RESEARCH, OSMOND TOOK MESCALINE TO EXPERIENCE ITS EFFECTS FOR HIMSELF.
GOING FOR A WALK WITH HIS WIFE, JANE, HE WAS STRICKEN BY FEAR AND PARANOIA.

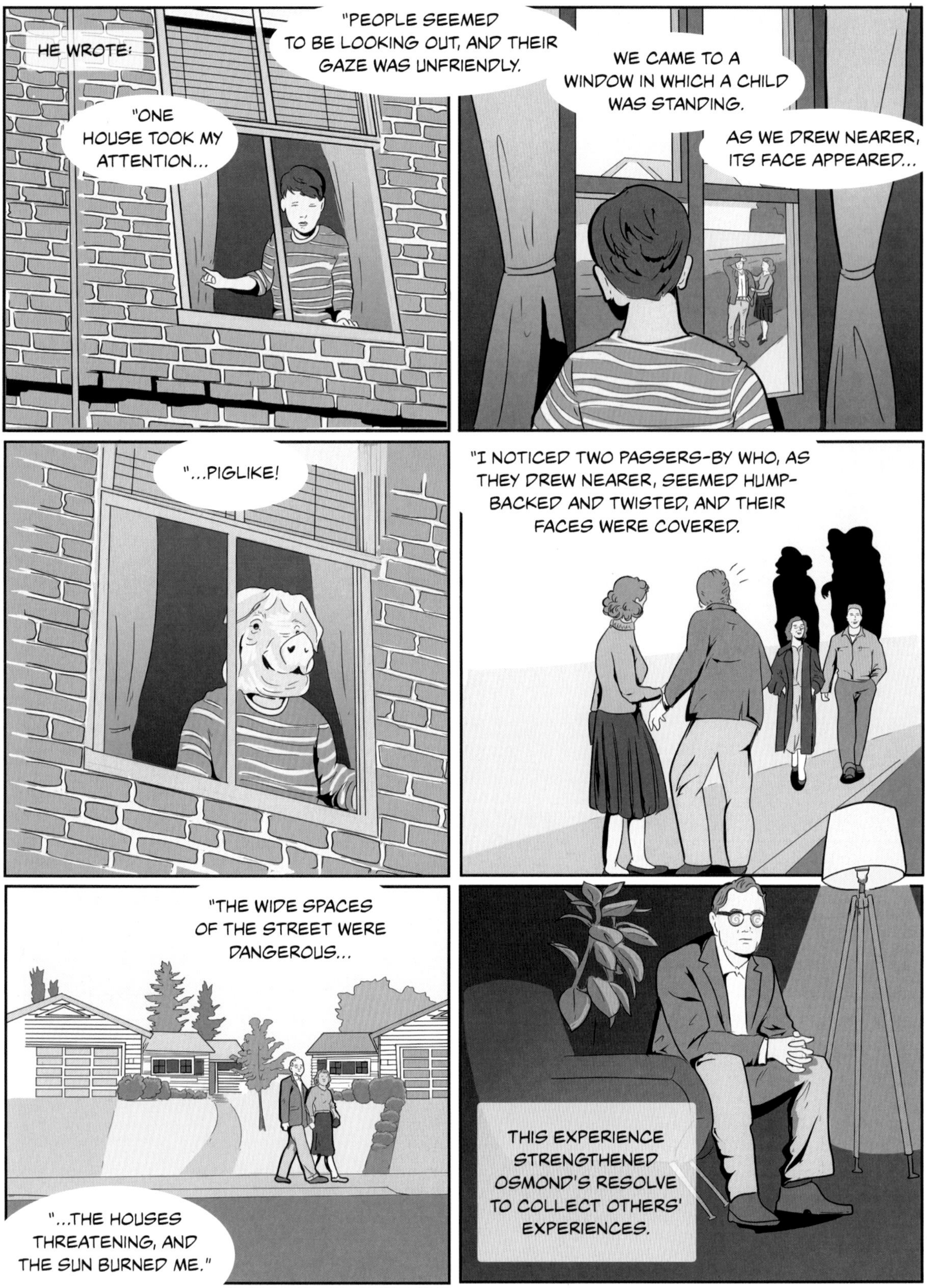

HE WROTE:
"PEOPLE SEEMED TO BE LOOKING OUT, AND THEIR GAZE WAS UNFRIENDLY.
"ONE HOUSE TOOK MY ATTENTION...
WE CAME TO A WINDOW IN WHICH A CHILD WAS STANDING.
AS WE DREW NEARER, ITS FACE APPEARED...
"...PIGLIKE!
"I NOTICED TWO PASSERS-BY WHO, AS THEY DREW NEARER, SEEMED HUMP-BACKED AND TWISTED, AND THEIR FACES WERE COVERED.
"THE WIDE SPACES OF THE STREET WERE DANGEROUS...
"...THE HOUSES THREATENING, AND THE SUN BURNED ME."
THIS EXPERIENCE STRENGTHENED OSMOND'S RESOLVE TO COLLECT OTHERS' EXPERIENCES.

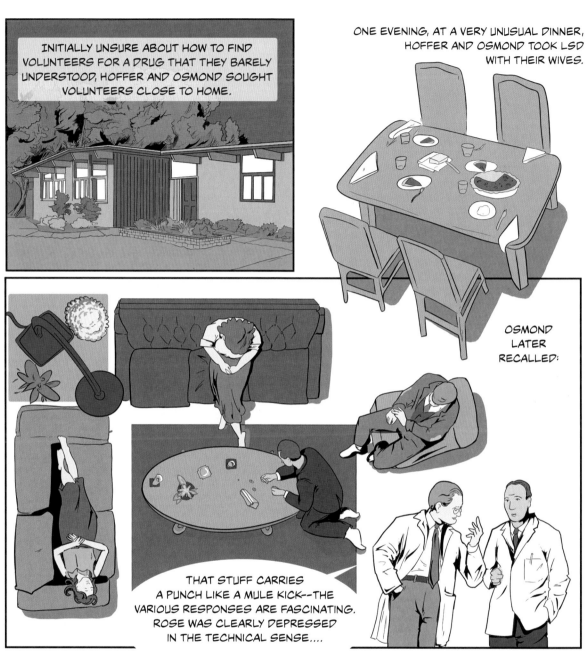

INITIALLY UNSURE ABOUT HOW TO FIND VOLUNTEERS FOR A DRUG THAT THEY BARELY UNDERSTOOD, HOFFER AND OSMOND SOUGHT VOLUNTEERS CLOSE TO HOME.

ONE EVENING, AT A VERY UNUSUAL DINNER, HOFFER AND OSMOND TOOK LSD WITH THEIR WIVES.

OSMOND LATER RECALLED:

THAT STUFF CARRIES A PUNCH LIKE A MULE KICK--THE VARIOUS RESPONSES ARE FASCINATING. ROSE WAS CLEARLY DEPRESSED IN THE TECHNICAL SENSE....

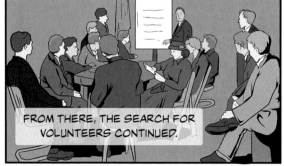

FROM THERE, THE SEARCH FOR VOLUNTEERS CONTINUED.

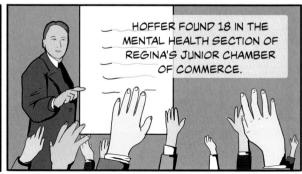

HOFFER FOUND 18 IN THE MENTAL HEALTH SECTION OF REGINA'S JUNIOR CHAMBER OF COMMERCE.

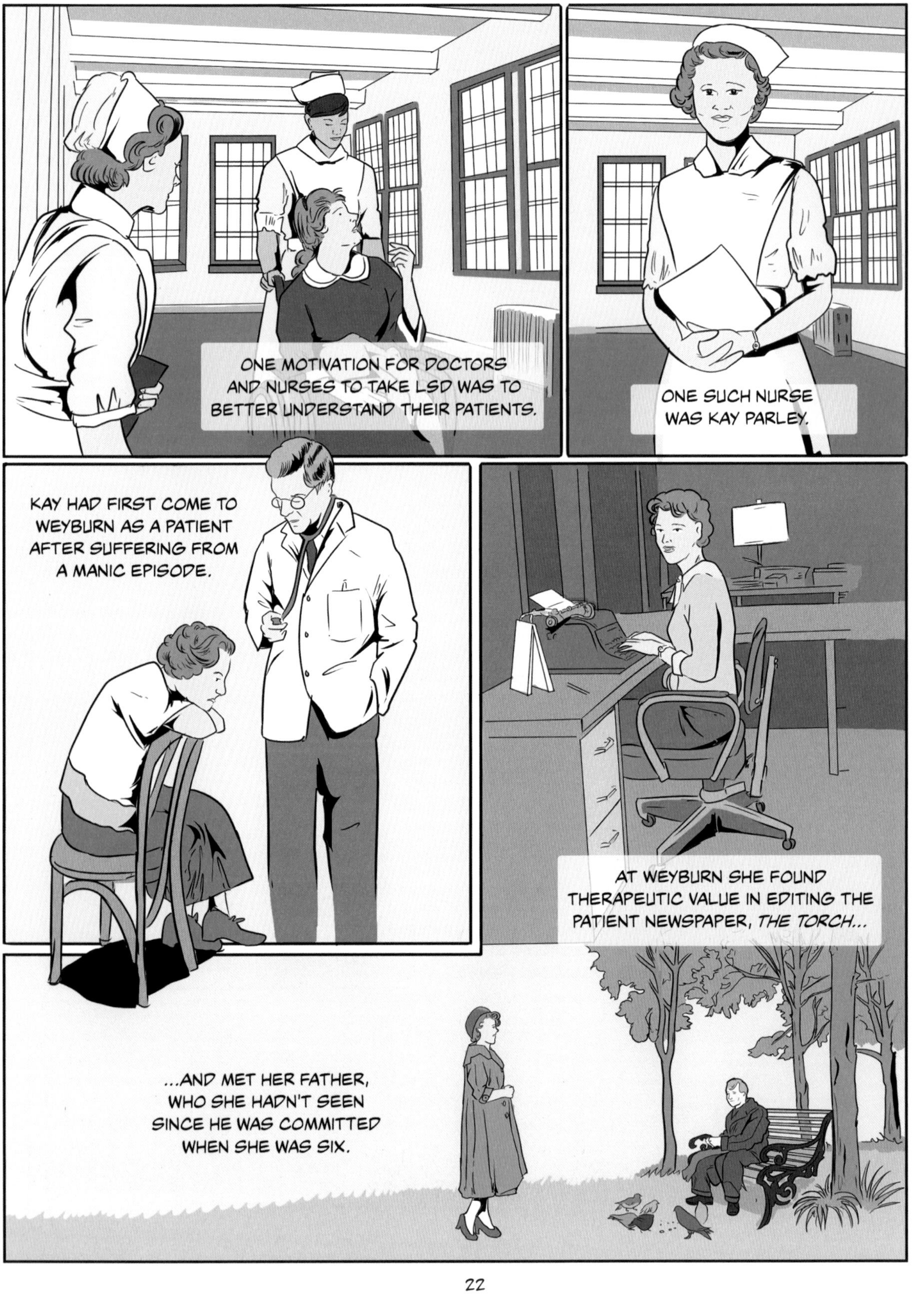
ONE MOTIVATION FOR DOCTORS AND NURSES TO TAKE LSD WAS TO BETTER UNDERSTAND THEIR PATIENTS.
ONE SUCH NURSE WAS KAY PARLEY.
KAY HAD FIRST COME TO WEYBURN AS A PATIENT AFTER SUFFERING FROM A MANIC EPISODE.
AT WEYBURN SHE FOUND THERAPEUTIC VALUE IN EDITING THE PATIENT NEWSPAPER, *THE TORCH*...
...AND MET HER FATHER, WHO SHE HADN'T SEEN SINCE HE WAS COMMITTED WHEN SHE WAS SIX.

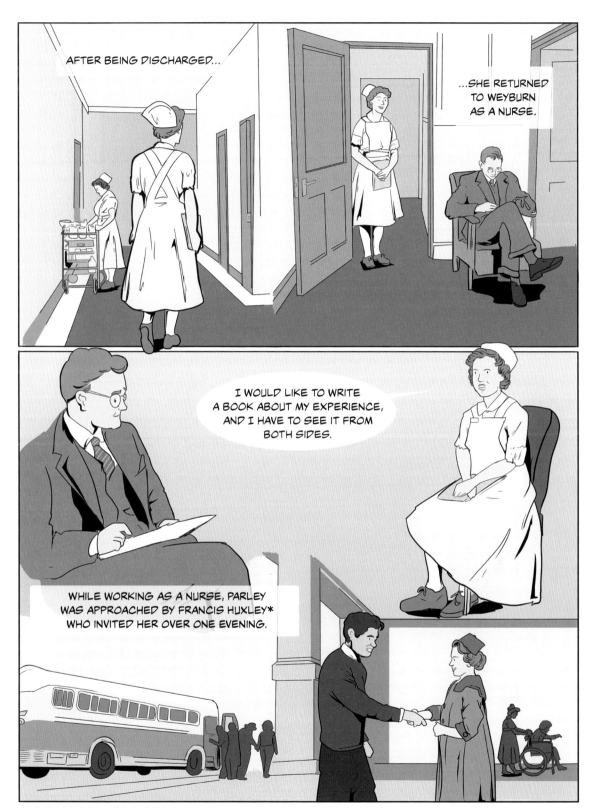

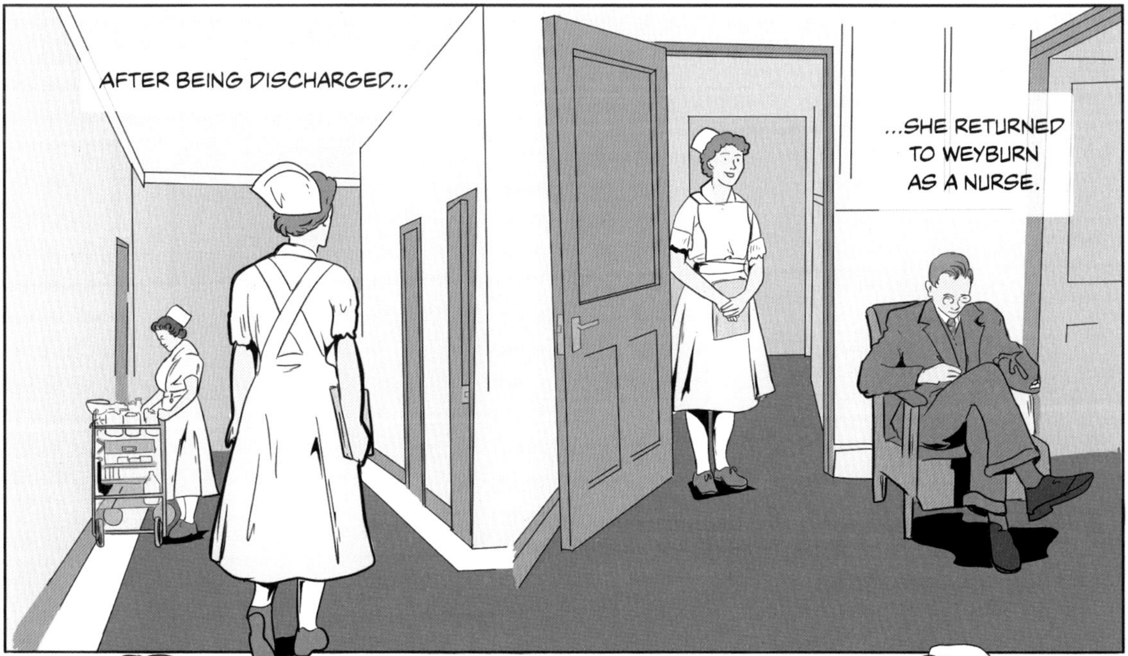
AFTER BEING DISCHARGED...
...SHE RETURNED TO WEYBURN AS A NURSE.

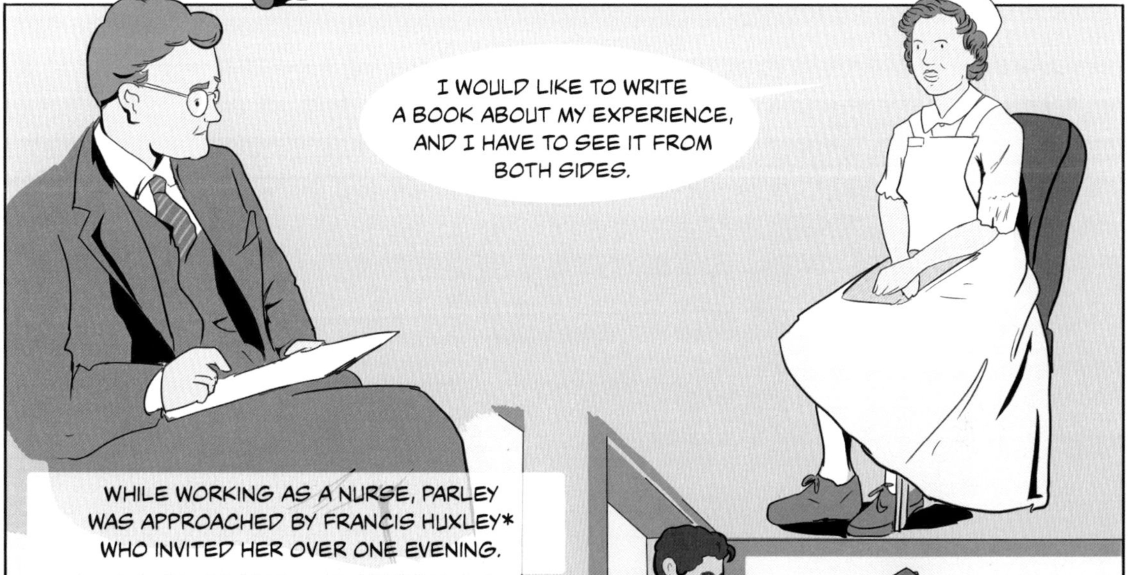
I WOULD LIKE TO WRITE A BOOK ABOUT MY EXPERIENCE, AND I HAVE TO SEE IT FROM BOTH SIDES.
WHILE WORKING AS A NURSE, PARLEY WAS APPROACHED BY FRANCIS HUXLEY* WHO INVITED HER OVER ONE EVENING.

*ALDOUS HUXLEY'S NEPHEW

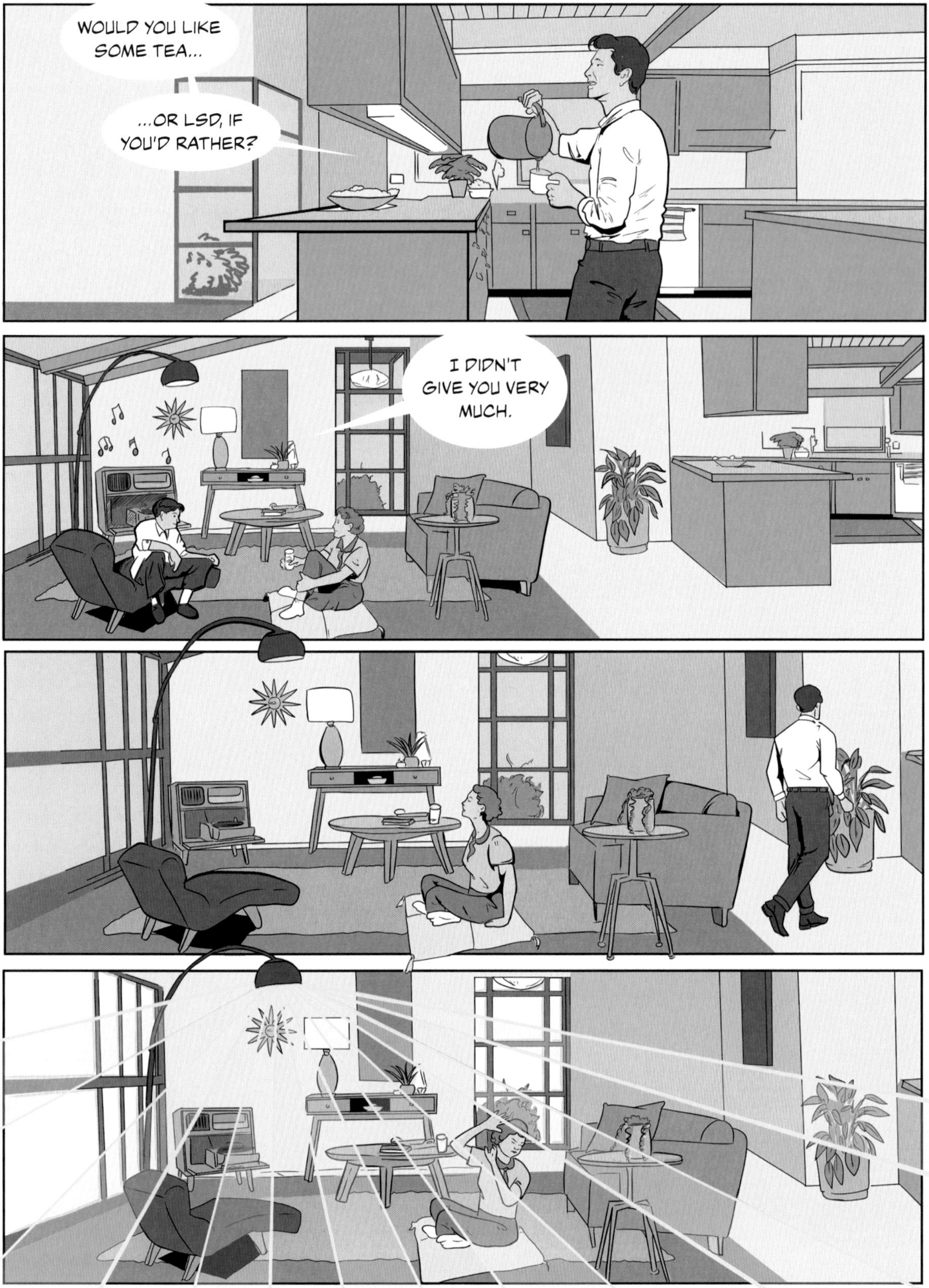
WOULD YOU LIKE SOME TEA...
...OR LSD, IF YOU'D RATHER?
I DIDN'T GIVE YOU VERY MUCH.

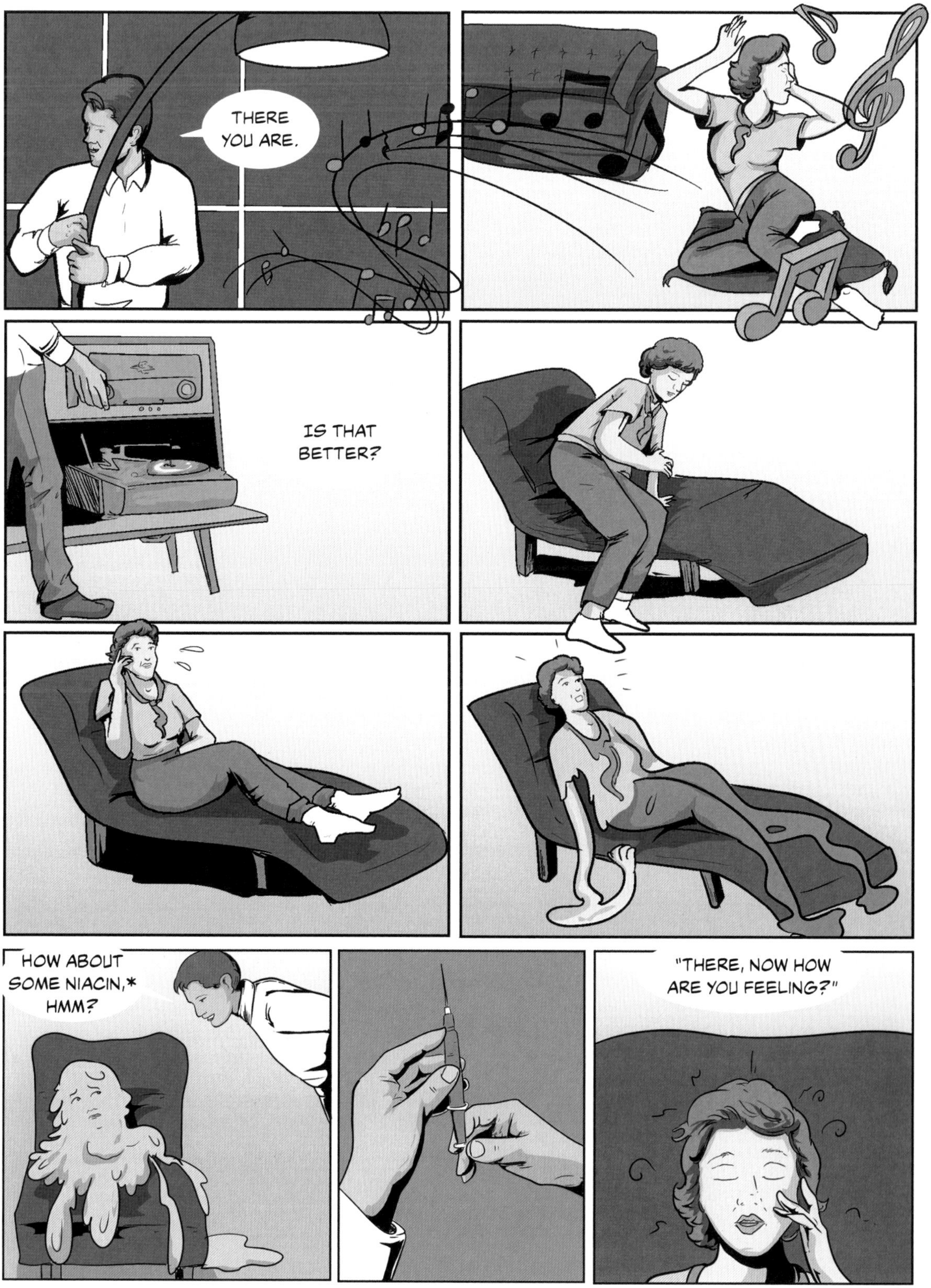
THERE YOU ARE.
IS THAT BETTER?
HOW ABOUT SOME NIACIN,* HMM?
"THERE, NOW HOW ARE YOU FEELING?"
*NIACIN REVERSES THE EFFECTS OF LSD.

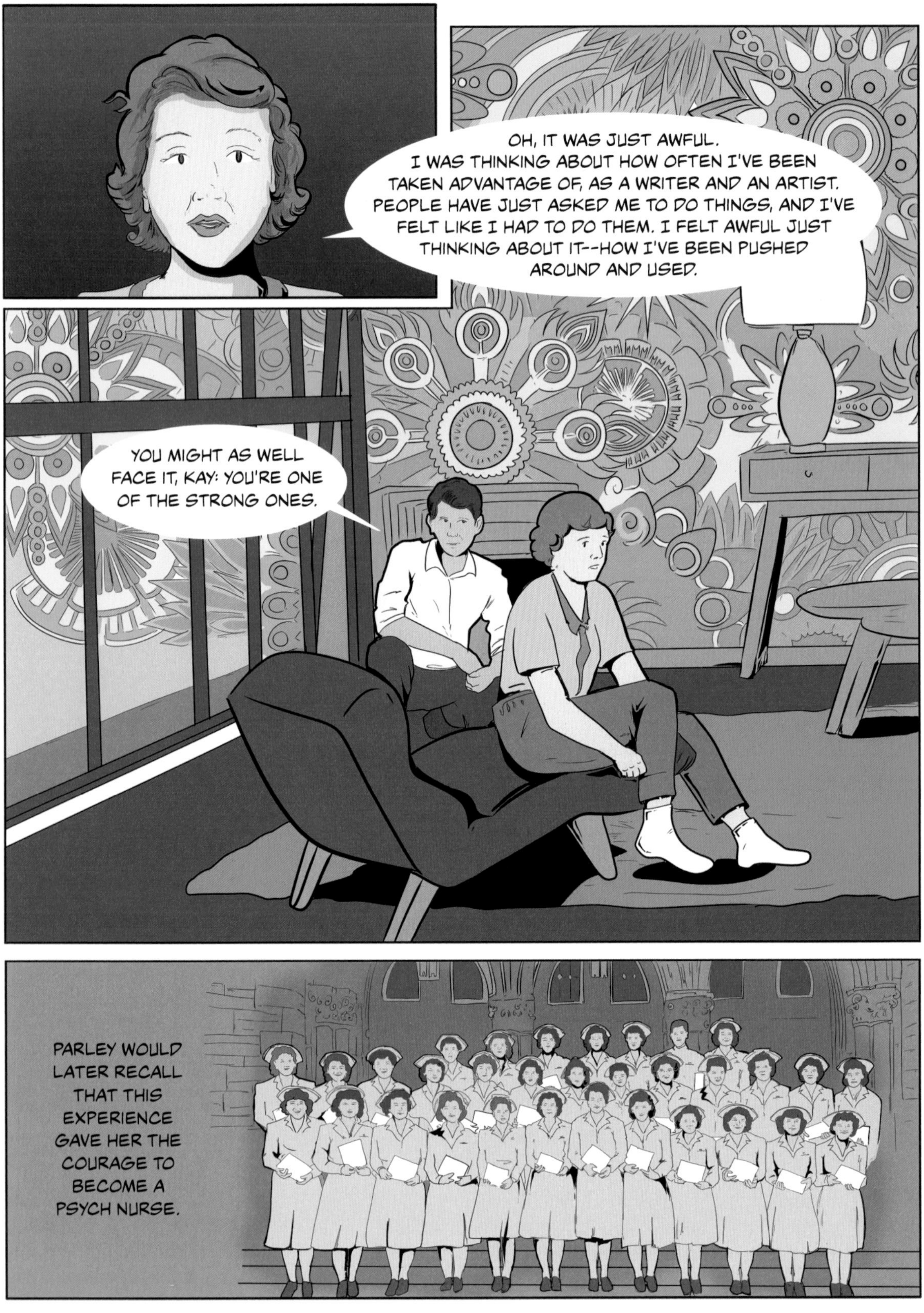
OH, IT WAS JUST AWFUL. I WAS THINKING ABOUT HOW OFTEN I'VE BEEN TAKEN ADVANTAGE OF, AS A WRITER AND AN ARTIST. PEOPLE HAVE JUST ASKED ME TO DO THINGS, AND I'VE FELT LIKE I HAD TO DO THEM. I FELT AWFUL JUST THINKING ABOUT IT--HOW I'VE BEEN PUSHED AROUND AND USED.
YOU MIGHT AS WELL FACE IT, KAY: YOU'RE ONE OF THE STRONG ONES.
PARLEY WOULD LATER RECALL THAT THIS EXPERIENCE GAVE HER THE COURAGE TO BECOME A PSYCH NURSE.

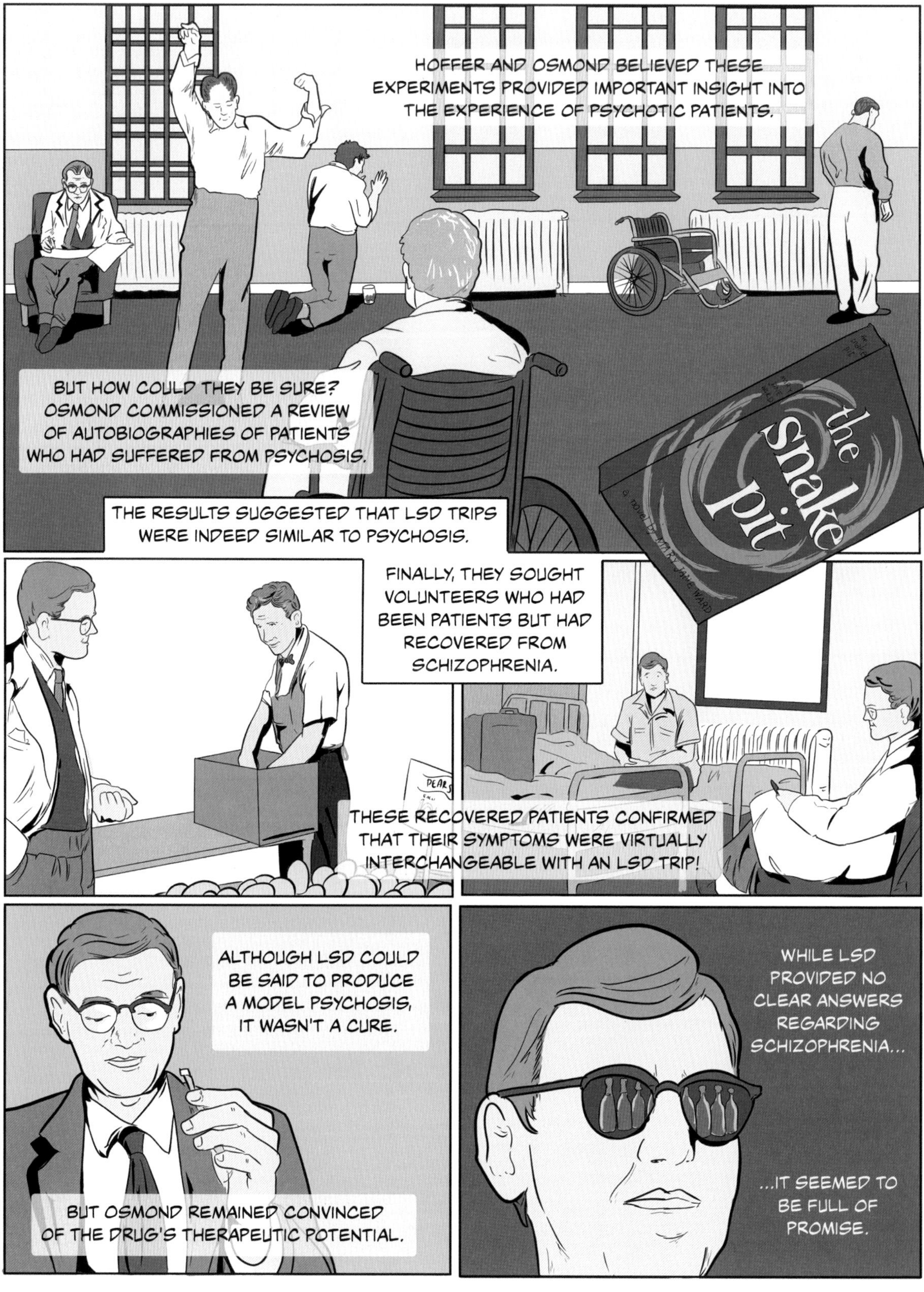
HOFFER AND OSMOND BELIEVED THESE EXPERIMENTS PROVIDED IMPORTANT INSIGHT INTO THE EXPERIENCE OF PSYCHOTIC PATIENTS.
BUT HOW COULD THEY BE SURE? OSMOND COMMISSIONED A REVIEW OF AUTOBIOGRAPHIES OF PATIENTS WHO HAD SUFFERED FROM PSYCHOSIS.
the snake pit
THE RESULTS SUGGESTED THAT LSD TRIPS WERE INDEED SIMILAR TO PSYCHOSIS.
FINALLY, THEY SOUGHT VOLUNTEERS WHO HAD BEEN PATIENTS BUT HAD RECOVERED FROM SCHIZOPHRENIA.
PEARS
THESE RECOVERED PATIENTS CONFIRMED THAT THEIR SYMPTOMS WERE VIRTUALLY INTERCHANGEABLE WITH AN LSD TRIP!
ALTHOUGH LSD COULD BE SAID TO PRODUCE A MODEL PSYCHOSIS, IT WASN'T A CURE.
BUT OSMOND REMAINED CONVINCED OF THE DRUG'S THERAPEUTIC POTENTIAL.
WHILE LSD PROVIDED NO CLEAR ANSWERS REGARDING SCHIZOPHRENIA...
...IT SEEMED TO BE FULL OF PROMISE.

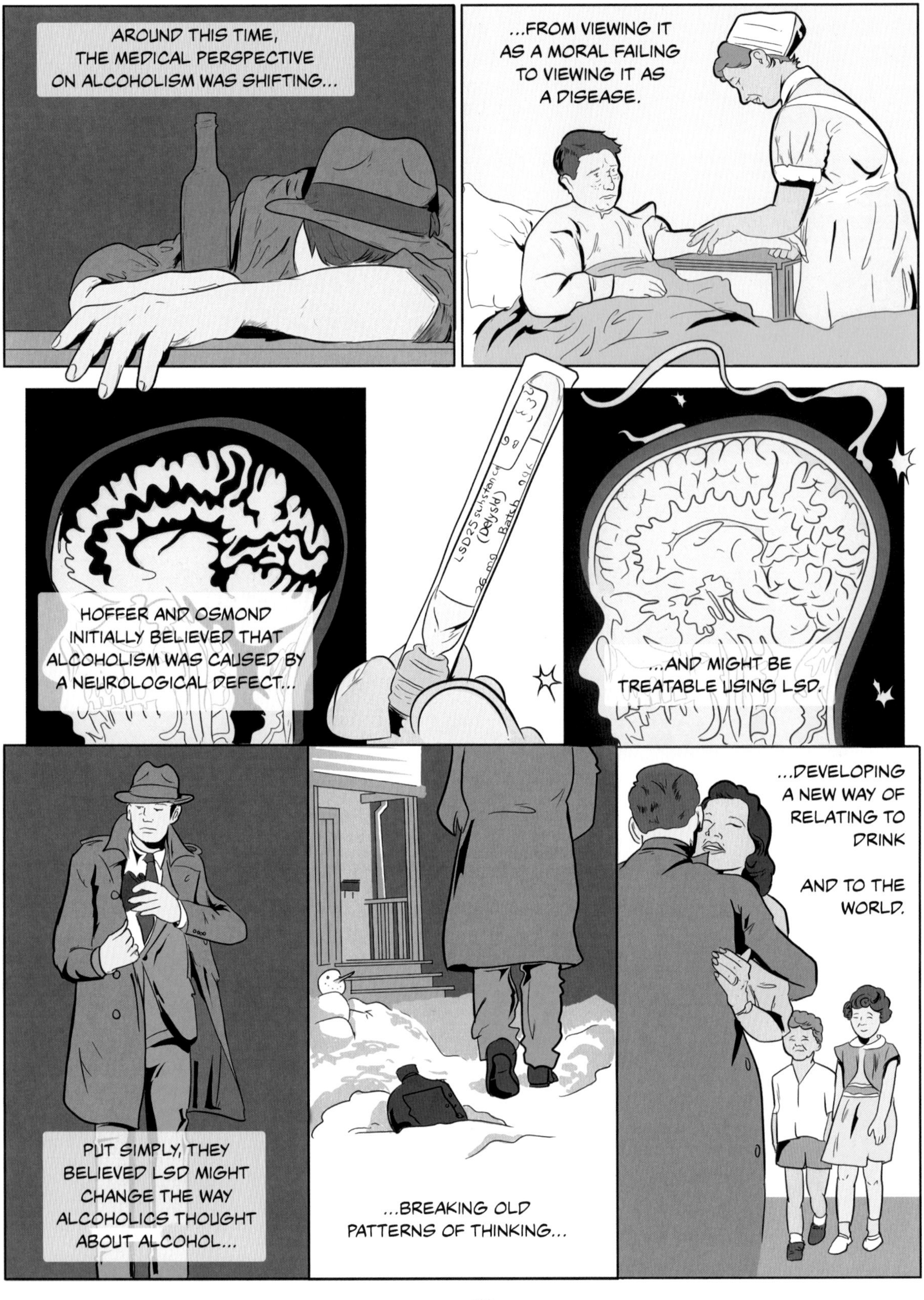
AROUND THIS TIME, THE MEDICAL PERSPECTIVE ON ALCOHOLISM WAS SHIFTING...
...FROM VIEWING IT AS A MORAL FAILING TO VIEWING IT AS A DISEASE.
HOFFER AND OSMOND INITIALLY BELIEVED THAT ALCOHOLISM WAS CAUSED BY A NEUROLOGICAL DEFECT...
LSD25 substance (Delysid) Batch 26 mg
...AND MIGHT BE TREATABLE USING LSD.
PUT SIMPLY, THEY BELIEVED LSD MIGHT CHANGE THE WAY ALCOHOLICS THOUGHT ABOUT ALCOHOL...
...BREAKING OLD PATTERNS OF THINKING...
...DEVELOPING A NEW WAY OF RELATING TO DRINK
AND TO THE WORLD.

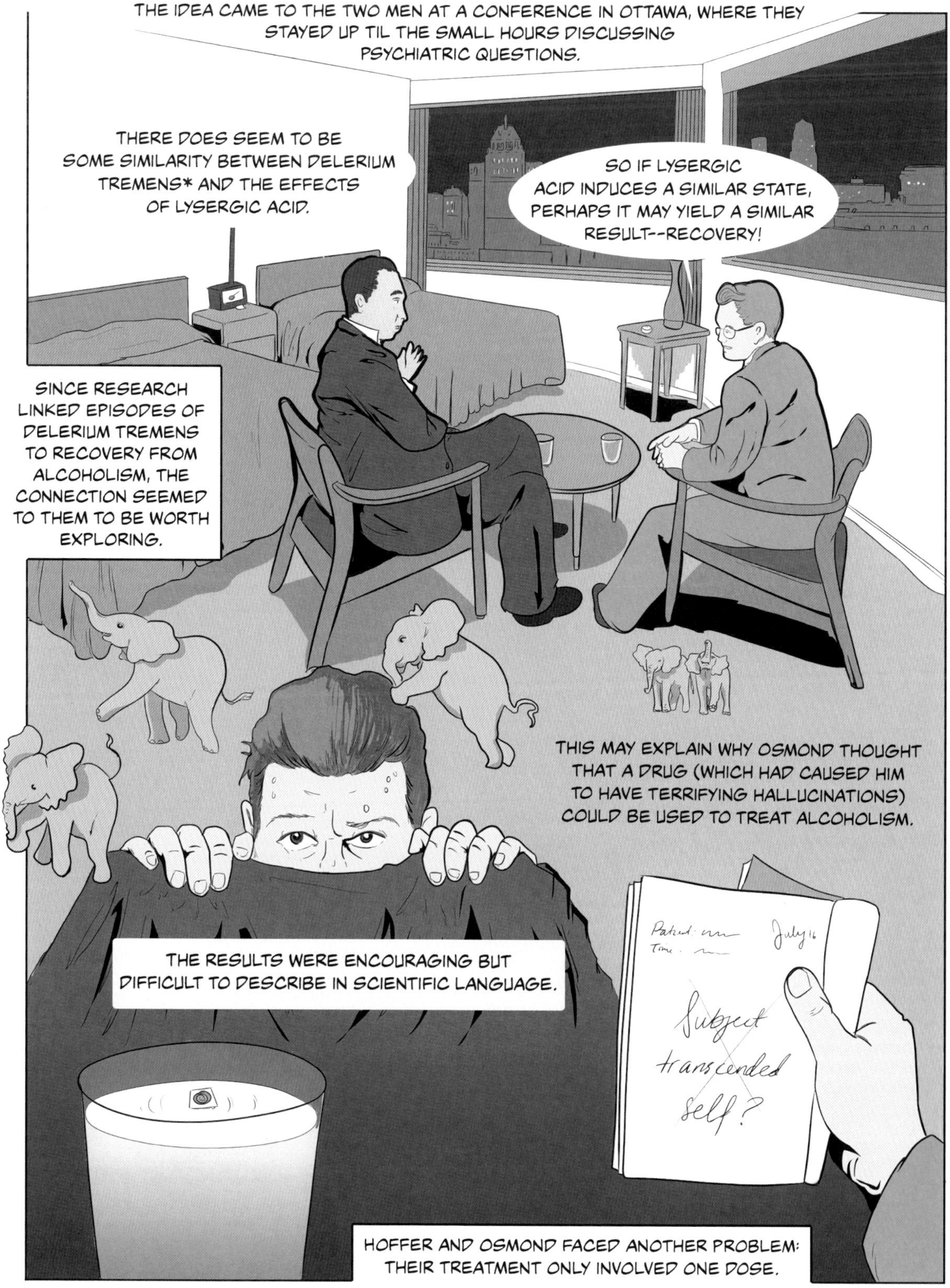
THE IDEA CAME TO THE TWO MEN AT A CONFERENCE IN OTTAWA, WHERE THEY STAYED UP TIL THE SMALL HOURS DISCUSSING PSYCHIATRIC QUESTIONS.
THERE DOES SEEM TO BE SOME SIMILARITY BETWEEN DELERIUM TREMENS* AND THE EFFECTS OF LYSERGIC ACID.
SO IF LYSERGIC ACID INDUCES A SIMILAR STATE, PERHAPS IT MAY YIELD A SIMILAR RESULT--RECOVERY!
SINCE RESEARCH LINKED EPISODES OF DELERIUM TREMENS TO RECOVERY FROM ALCOHOLISM, THE CONNECTION SEEMED TO THEM TO BE WORTH EXPLORING.
THIS MAY EXPLAIN WHY OSMOND THOUGHT THAT A DRUG (WHICH HAD CAUSED HIM TO HAVE TERRIFYING HALLUCINATIONS) COULD BE USED TO TREAT ALCOHOLISM.
THE RESULTS WERE ENCOURAGING BUT DIFFICULT TO DESCRIBE IN SCIENTIFIC LANGUAGE.
July 16
Subject transcended self?
HOFFER AND OSMOND FACED ANOTHER PROBLEM: THEIR TREATMENT ONLY INVOLVED ONE DOSE.

*ALCOHOL WITHDRAWAL

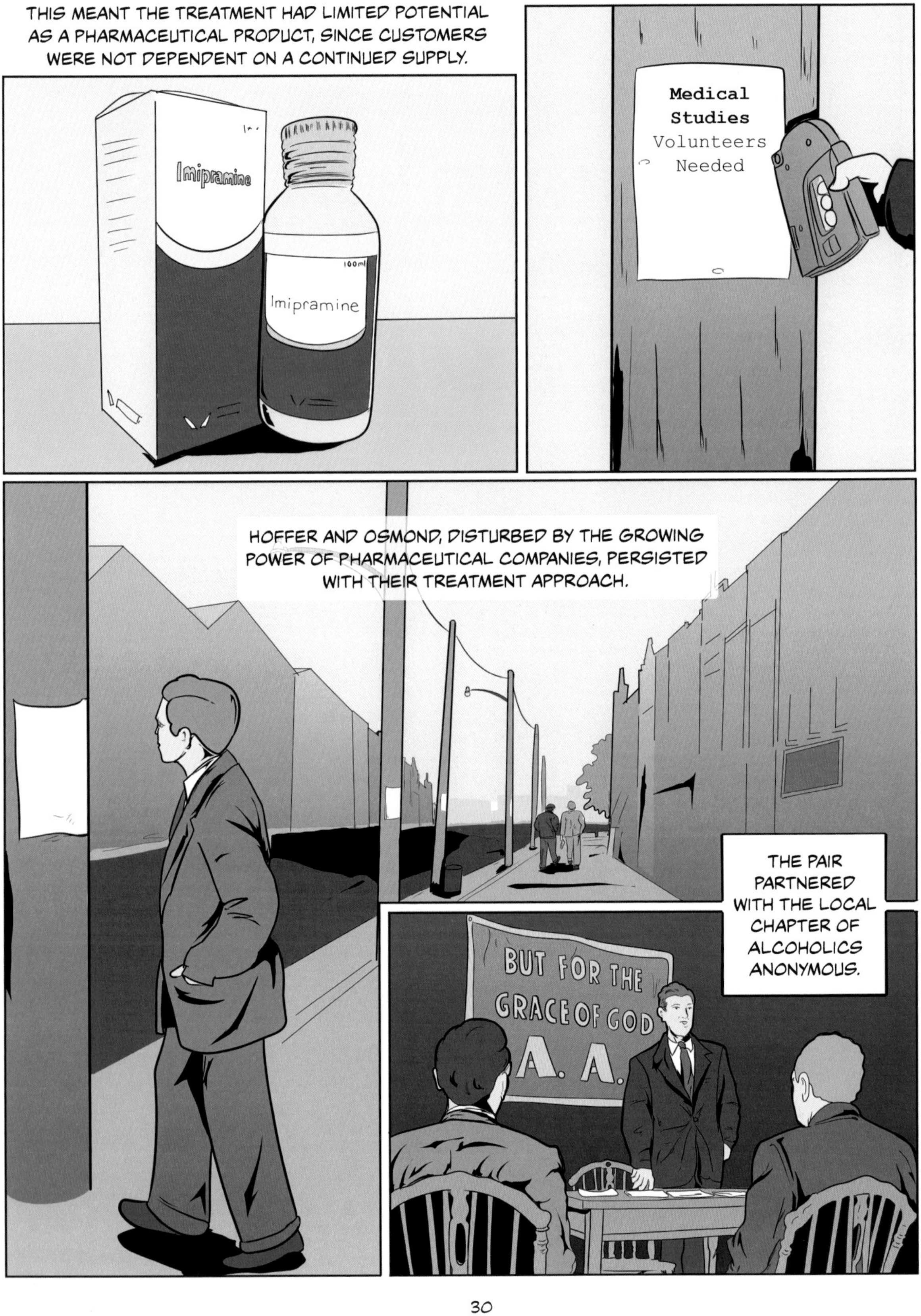
THIS MEANT THE TREATMENT HAD LIMITED POTENTIAL AS A PHARMACEUTICAL PRODUCT, SINCE CUSTOMERS WERE NOT DEPENDENT ON A CONTINUED SUPPLY.
Imipramine
100ml
Imipramine
Medical Studies
Volunteers Needed
HOFFER AND OSMOND, DISTURBED BY THE GROWING POWER OF PHARMACEUTICAL COMPANIES, PERSISTED WITH THEIR TREATMENT APPROACH.
THE PAIR PARTNERED WITH THE LOCAL CHAPTER OF ALCOHOLICS ANONYMOUS.
BUT FOR THE GRACE OF GOD
A. A.

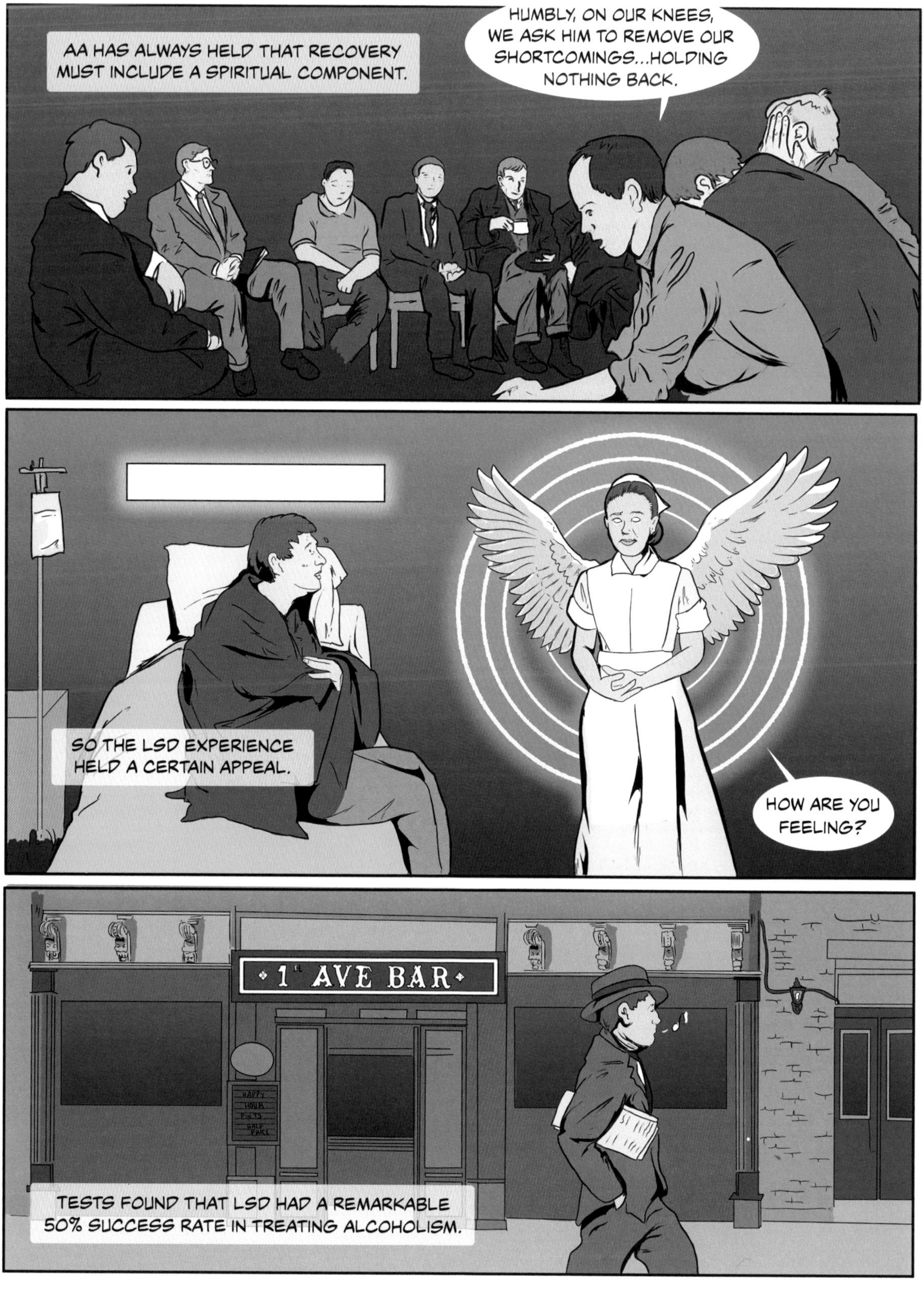
AA HAS ALWAYS HELD THAT RECOVERY MUST INCLUDE A SPIRITUAL COMPONENT.
HUMBLY, ON OUR KNEES, WE ASK HIM TO REMOVE OUR SHORTCOMINGS...HOLDING NOTHING BACK.
SO THE LSD EXPERIENCE HELD A CERTAIN APPEAL.
HOW ARE YOU FEELING?
1st AVE BAR
TESTS FOUND THAT LSD HAD A REMARKABLE 50% SUCCESS RATE IN TREATING ALCOHOLISM.

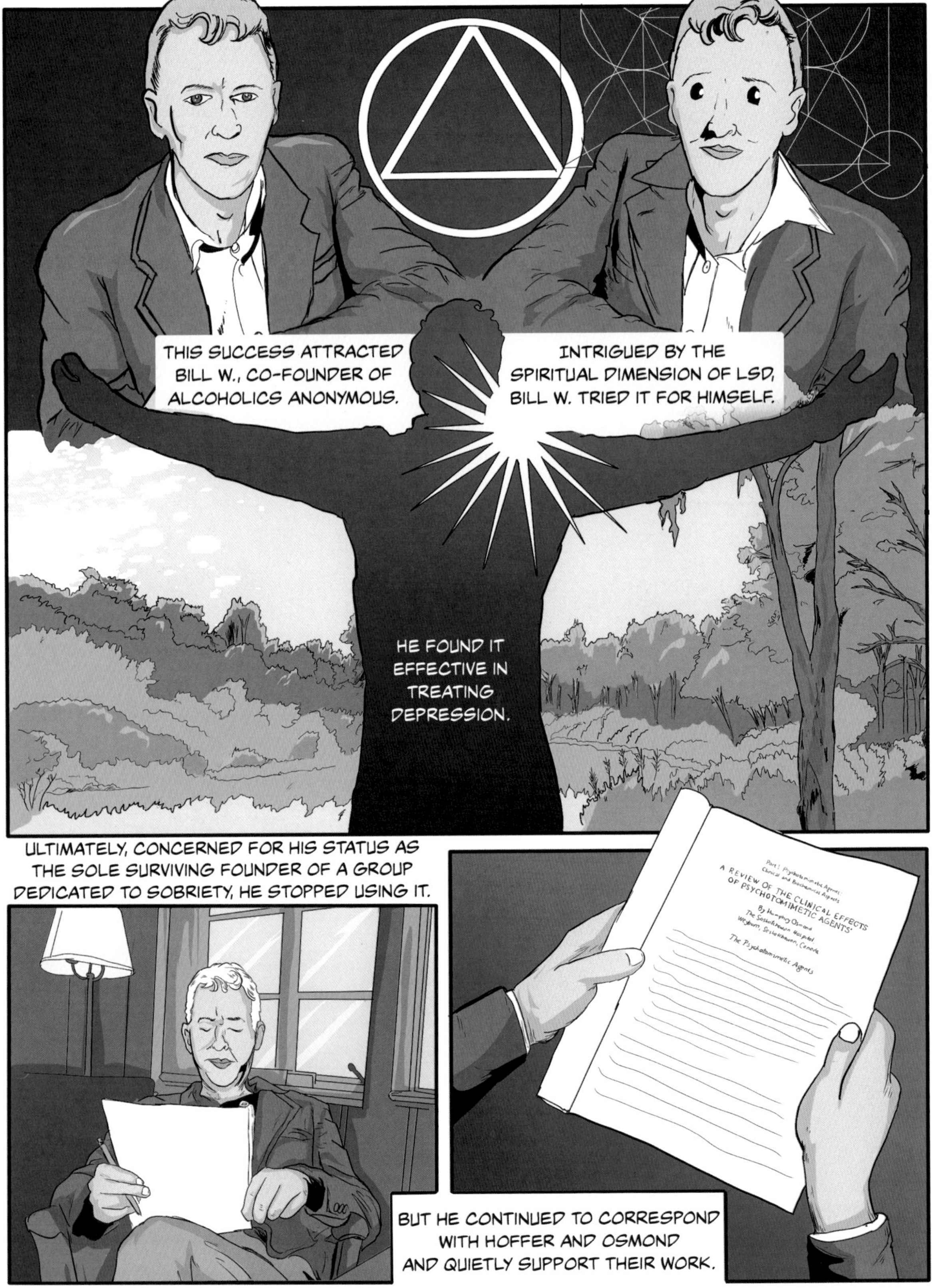
THIS SUCCESS ATTRACTED BILL W., CO-FOUNDER OF ALCOHOLICS ANONYMOUS.
INTRIGUED BY THE SPIRITUAL DIMENSION OF LSD, BILL W. TRIED IT FOR HIMSELF.
HE FOUND IT EFFECTIVE IN TREATING DEPRESSION.
ULTIMATELY, CONCERNED FOR HIS STATUS AS THE SOLE SURVIVING FOUNDER OF A GROUP DEDICATED TO SOBRIETY, HE STOPPED USING IT.
A REVIEW OF THE CLINICAL EFFECTS OF PSYCHOTOMIMETIC AGENTS'
The Psychotomimetic Agents
BUT HE CONTINUED TO CORRESPOND WITH HOFFER AND OSMOND AND QUIETLY SUPPORT THEIR WORK.

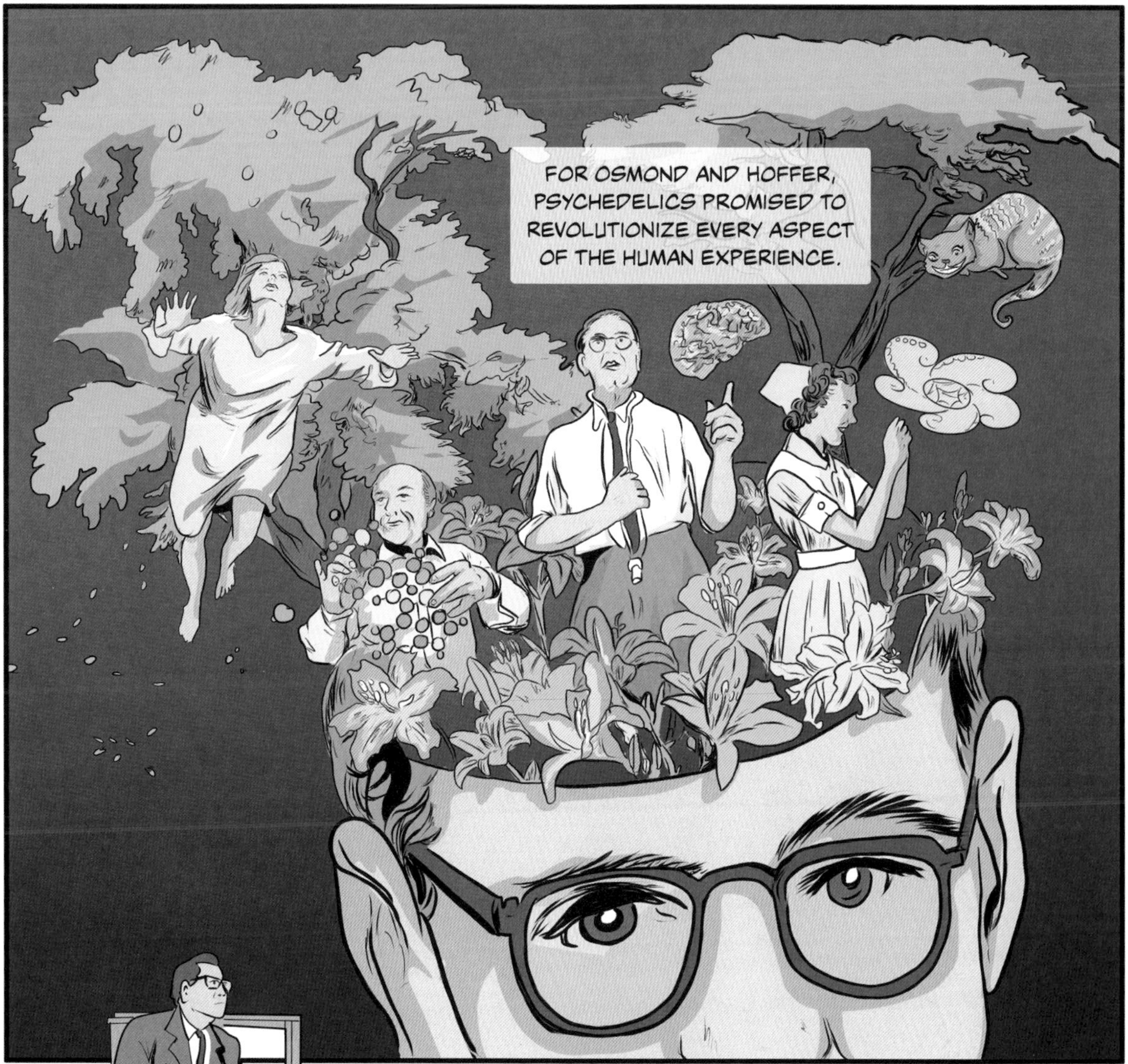
FOR OSMOND AND HOFFER, PSYCHEDELICS PROMISED TO REVOLUTIONIZE EVERY ASPECT OF THE HUMAN EXPERIENCE.

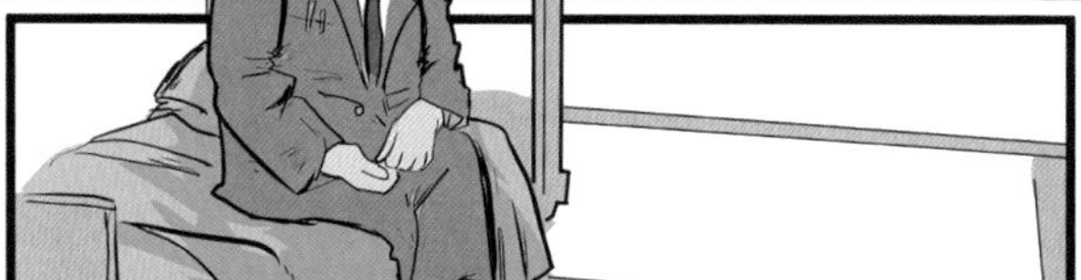

AMID A FIERCE PROFESSIONAL DEBATE ABOUT THE VALUE OF LONG-TERM MENTAL HEALTH INSTITUTIONS, THEY INVITED THE ARCHITECT KIYOSHI IZUMI AND HIS WIFE, AMY, TO VISIT WEYBURN.

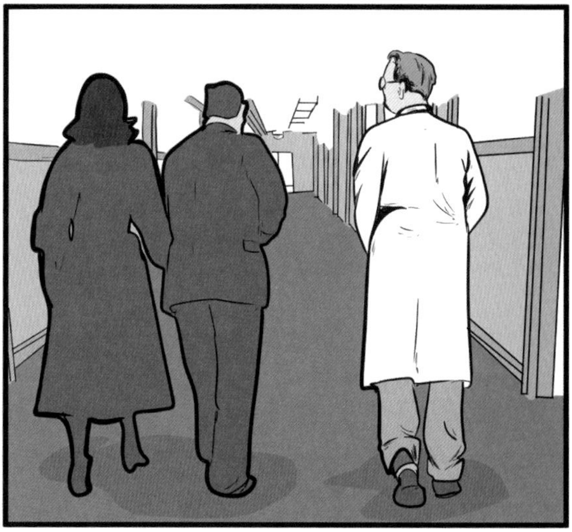

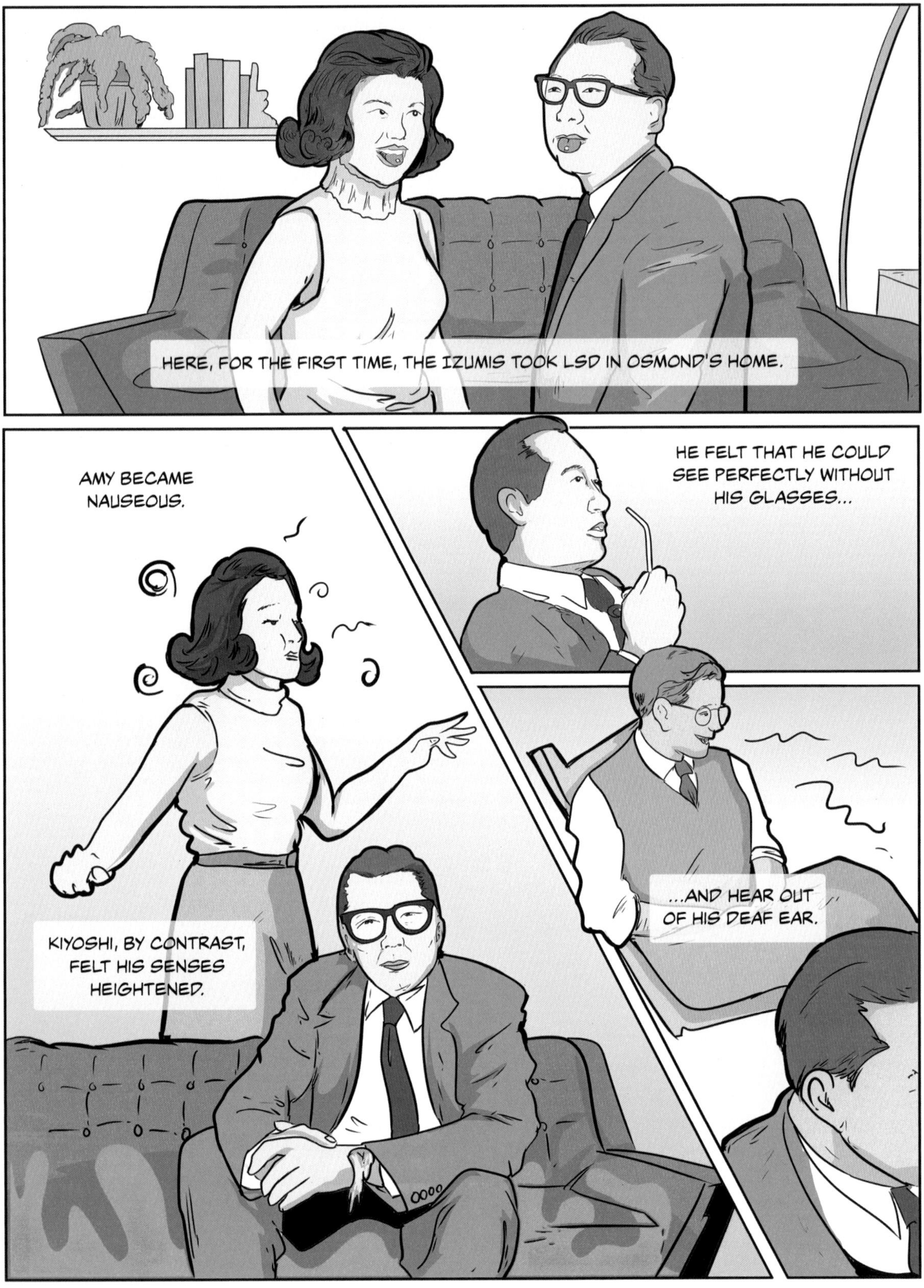
HERE, FOR THE FIRST TIME, THE IZUMIS TOOK LSD IN OSMOND'S HOME.
AMY BECAME NAUSEOUS.
HE FELT THAT HE COULD SEE PERFECTLY WITHOUT HIS GLASSES...
...AND HEAR OUT OF HIS DEAF EAR.
KIYOSHI, BY CONTRAST, FELT HIS SENSES HEIGHTENED.

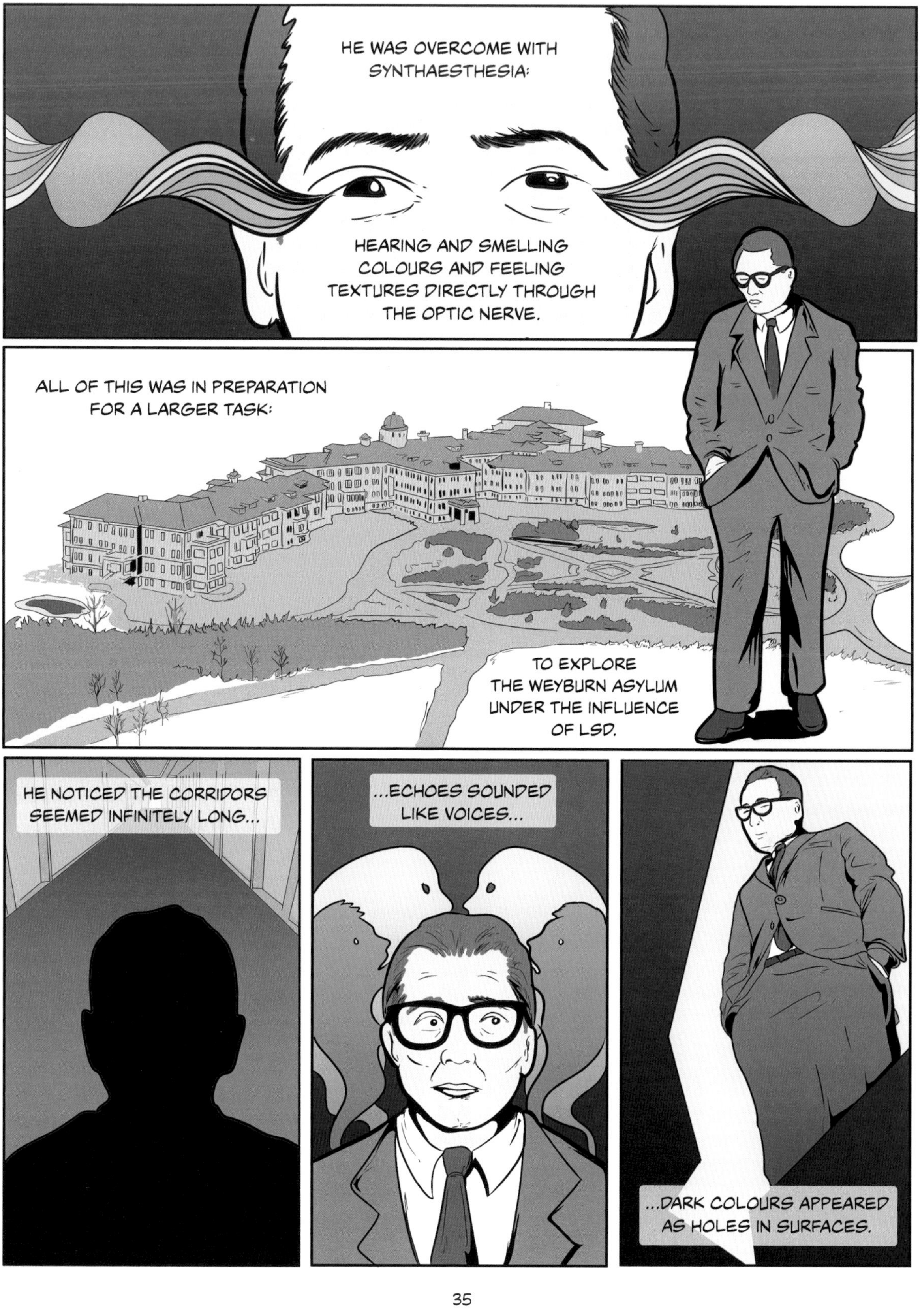
HE WAS OVERCOME WITH SYNTHAESTHESIA:
HEARING AND SMELLING COLOURS AND FEELING TEXTURES DIRECTLY THROUGH THE OPTIC NERVE.
ALL OF THIS WAS IN PREPARATION FOR A LARGER TASK:
TO EXPLORE THE WEYBURN ASYLUM UNDER THE INFLUENCE OF LSD.
HE NOTICED THE CORRIDORS SEEMED INFINITELY LONG...
...ECHOES SOUNDED LIKE VOICES...
...DARK COLOURS APPEARED AS HOLES IN SURFACES.

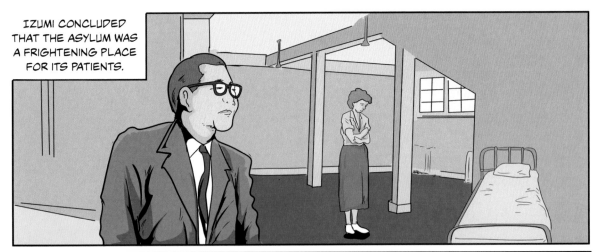

IZUMI CONCLUDED THAT THE ASYLUM WAS A FRIGHTENING PLACE FOR ITS PATIENTS.

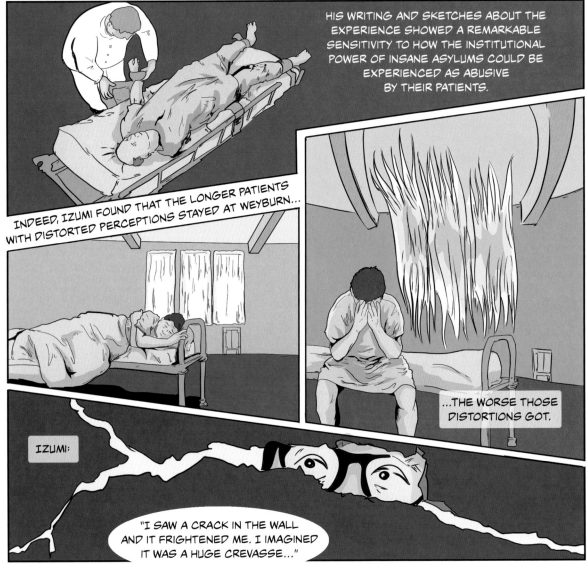

HIS WRITING AND SKETCHES ABOUT THE EXPERIENCE SHOWED A REMARKABLE SENSITIVITY TO HOW THE INSTITUTIONAL POWER OF INSANE ASYLUMS COULD BE EXPERIENCED AS ABUSIVE BY THEIR PATIENTS.

INDEED, IZUMI FOUND THAT THE LONGER PATIENTS WITH DISTORTED PERCEPTIONS STAYED AT WEYBURN...

...THE WORSE THOSE DISTORTIONS GOT.

IZUMI:

"I SAW A CRACK IN THE WALL AND IT FRIGHTENED ME. I IMAGINED IT WAS A HUGE CREVASSE..."

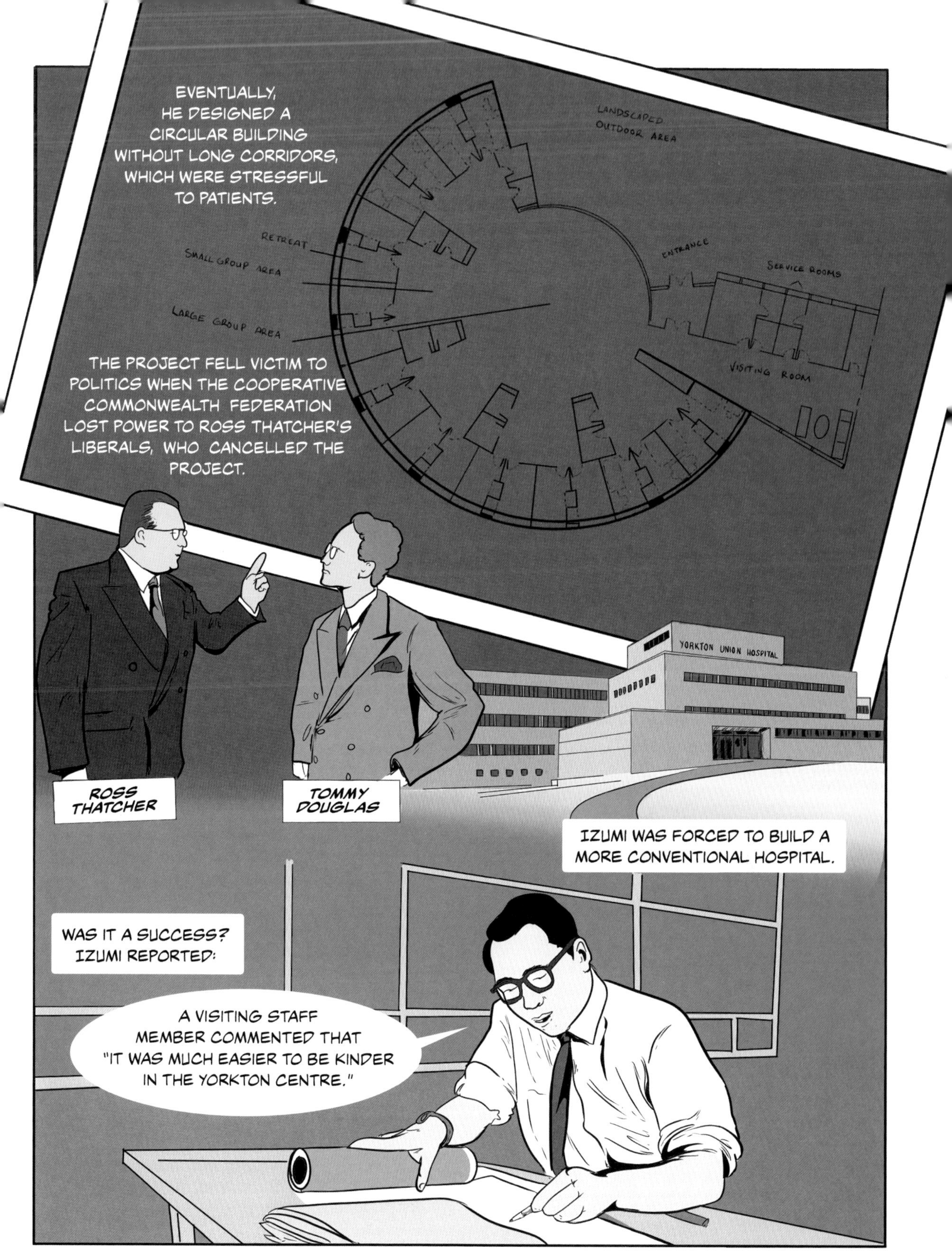
EVENTUALLY, HE DESIGNED A CIRCULAR BUILDING WITHOUT LONG CORRIDORS, WHICH WERE STRESSFUL TO PATIENTS.
LANDSCAPED OUTDOOR AREA
RETREAT
SMALL GROUP AREA
LARGE GROUP AREA
ENTRANCE
SERVICE ROOMS
VISITING ROOM
THE PROJECT FELL VICTIM TO POLITICS WHEN THE COOPERATIVE COMMONWEALTH FEDERATION LOST POWER TO ROSS THATCHER'S LIBERALS, WHO CANCELLED THE PROJECT.
ROSS THATCHER
TOMMY DOUGLAS
YORKTON UNION HOSPITAL
IZUMI WAS FORCED TO BUILD A MORE CONVENTIONAL HOSPITAL.
WAS IT A SUCCESS? IZUMI REPORTED:
A VISITING STAFF MEMBER COMMENTED THAT "IT WAS MUCH EASIER TO BE KINDER IN THE YORKTON CENTRE."

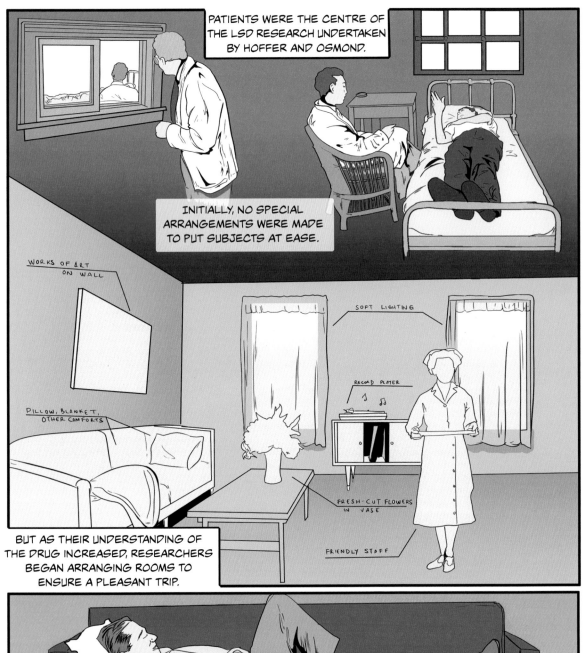

PATIENTS WERE THE CENTRE OF THE LSD RESEARCH UNDERTAKEN BY HOFFER AND OSMOND.

INITIALLY, NO SPECIAL ARRANGEMENTS WERE MADE TO PUT SUBJECTS AT EASE.

WORKS OF ART ON WALL

PILLOW, BLANKET, OTHER COMFORTS

SOFT LIGHTING

RECORD PLAYER

FRESH-CUT FLOWERS IN VASE

FRIENDLY STAFF

BUT AS THEIR UNDERSTANDING OF THE DRUG INCREASED, RESEARCHERS BEGAN ARRANGING ROOMS TO ENSURE A PLEASANT TRIP.

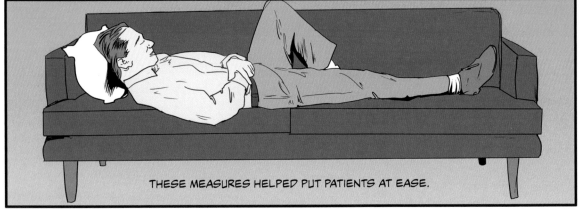

THESE MEASURES HELPED PUT PATIENTS AT EASE.

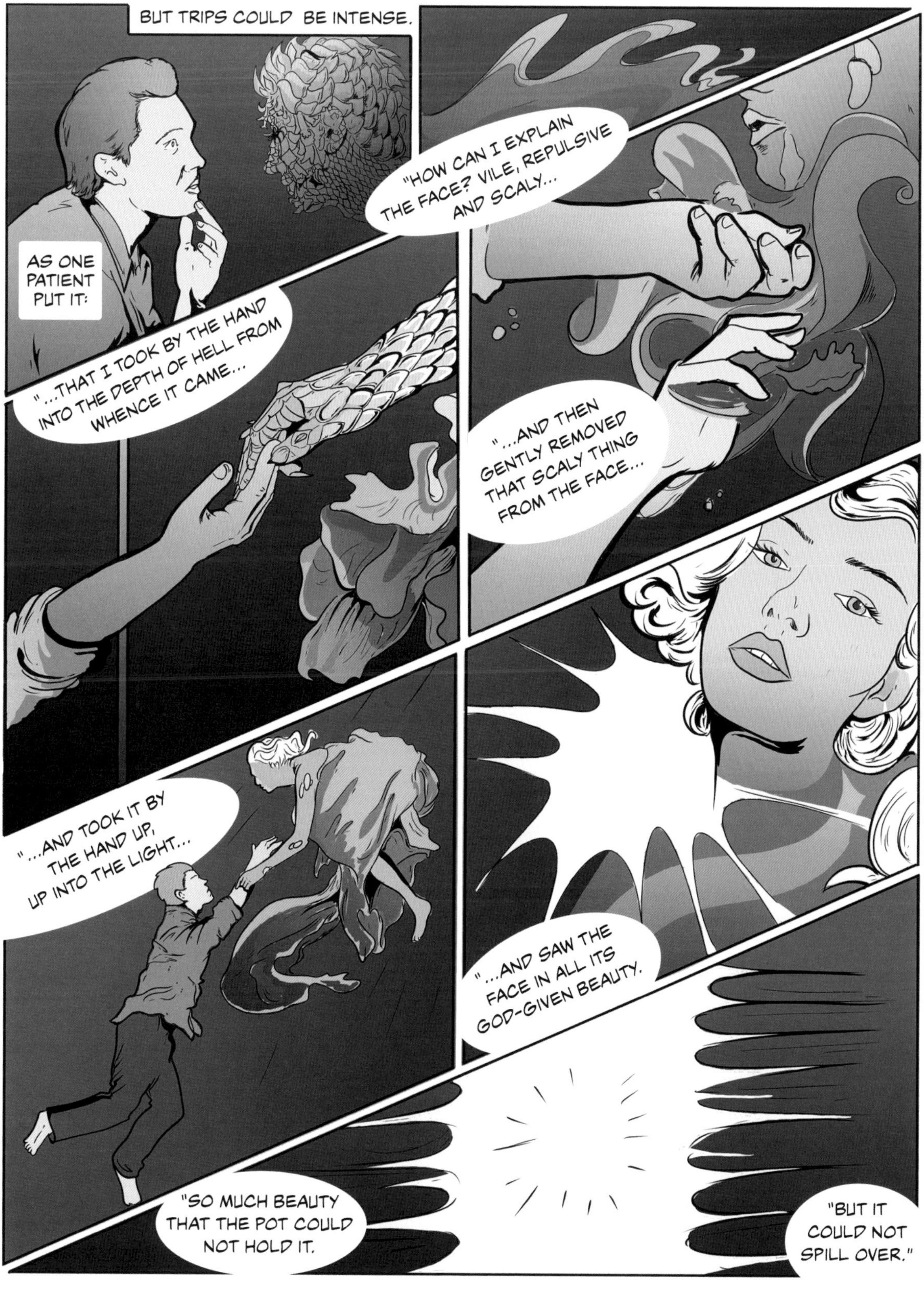
BUT TRIPS COULD BE INTENSE.
AS ONE PATIENT PUT IT:
"HOW CAN I EXPLAIN THE FACE? VILE, REPULSIVE AND SCALY...
"...THAT I TOOK BY THE HAND INTO THE DEPTH OF HELL FROM WHENCE IT CAME...
"...AND THEN GENTLY REMOVED THAT SCALY THING FROM THE FACE...
"...AND TOOK IT BY THE HAND UP, UP INTO THE LIGHT...
"...AND SAW THE FACE IN ALL ITS GOD-GIVEN BEAUTY.
"SO MUCH BEAUTY THAT THE POT COULD NOT HOLD IT.
"BUT IT COULD NOT SPILL OVER."

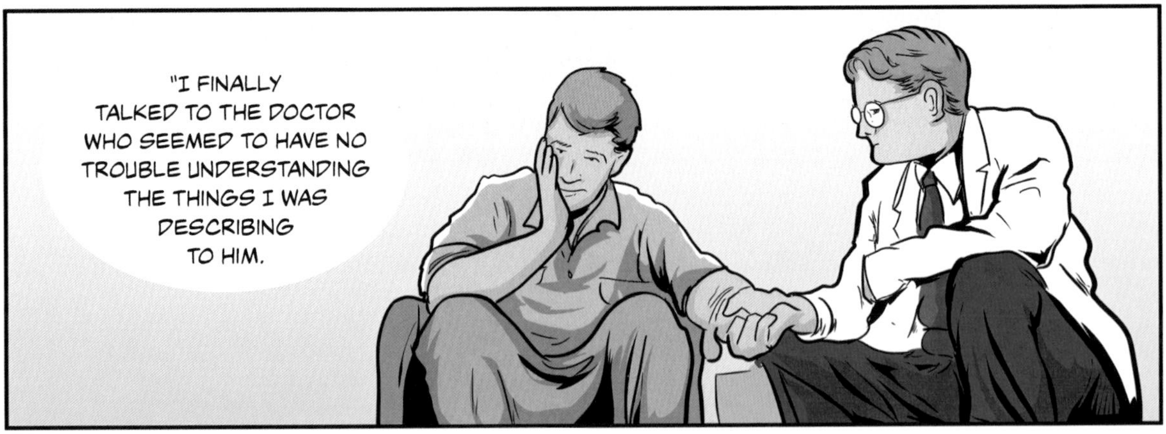
"I FINALLY TALKED TO THE DOCTOR WHO SEEMED TO HAVE NO TROUBLE UNDERSTANDING THE THINGS I WAS DESCRIBING TO HIM.

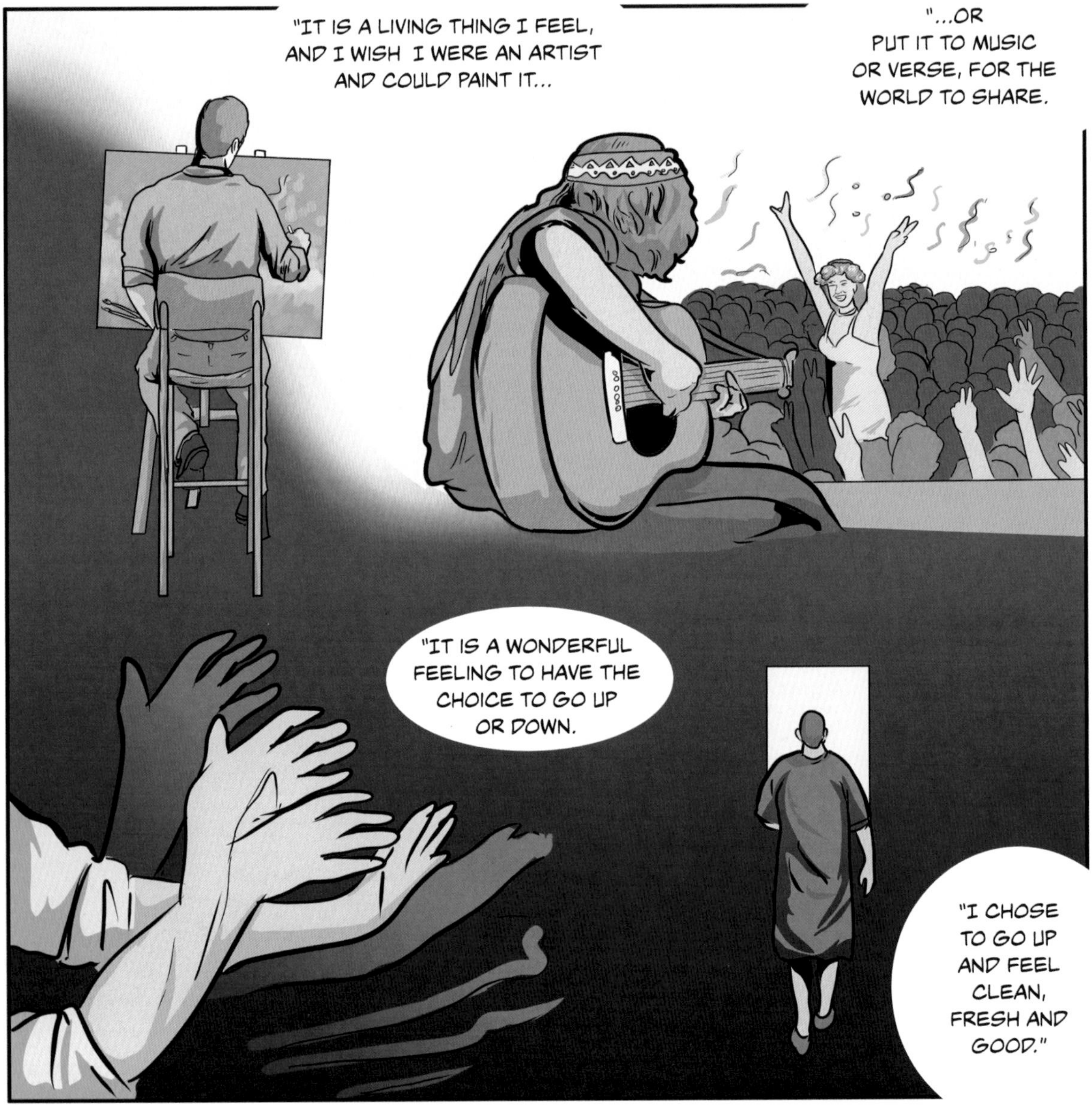
"IT IS A LIVING THING I FEEL, AND I WISH I WERE AN ARTIST AND COULD PAINT IT...
"...OR PUT IT TO MUSIC OR VERSE, FOR THE WORLD TO SHARE.
"IT IS A WONDERFUL FEELING TO HAVE THE CHOICE TO GO UP OR DOWN.
"I CHOSE TO GO UP AND FEEL CLEAN, FRESH AND GOOD."

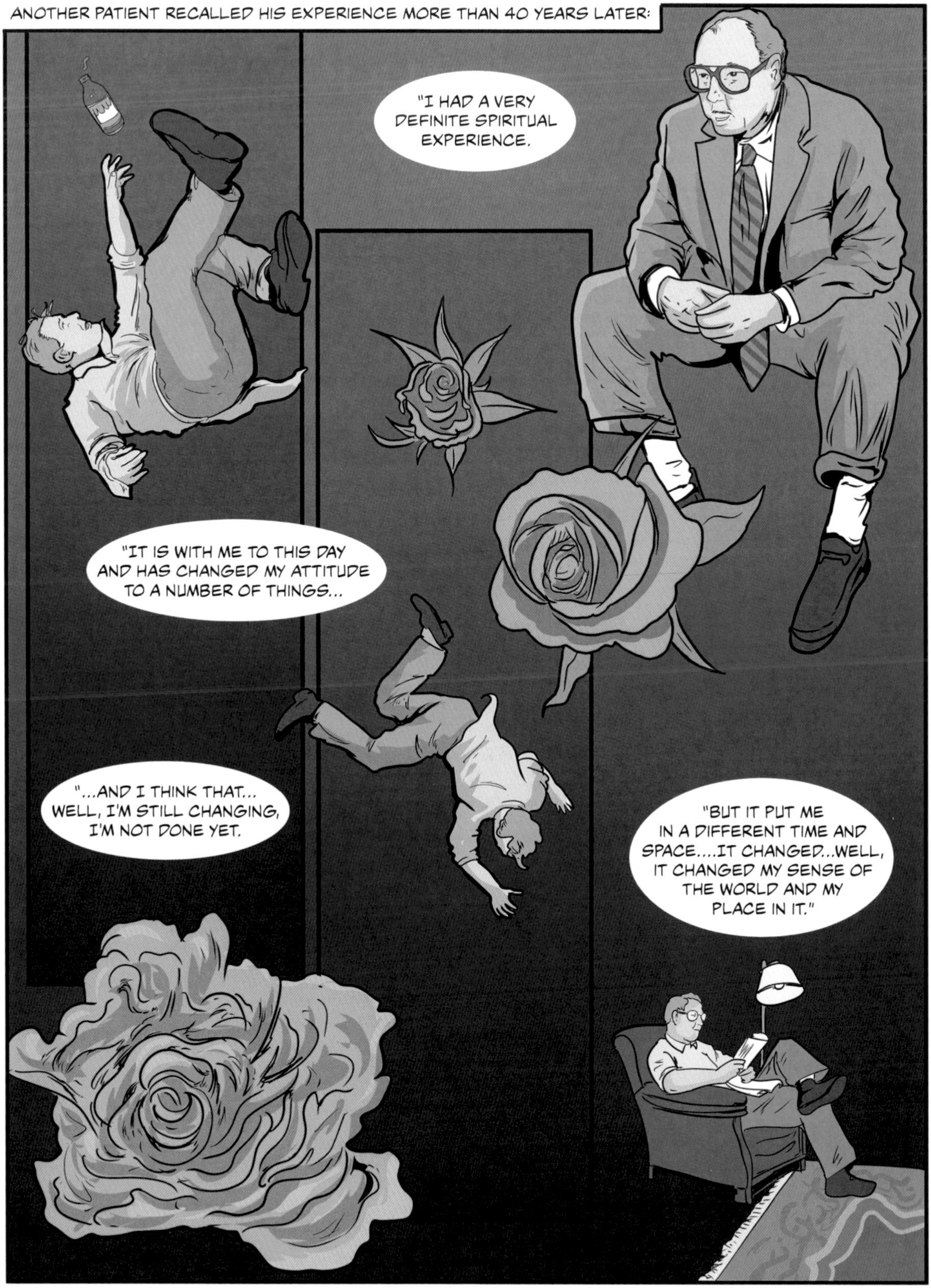
ANOTHER PATIENT RECALLED HIS EXPERIENCE MORE THAN 40 YEARS LATER:
"I HAD A VERY DEFINITE SPIRITUAL EXPERIENCE.
"IT IS WITH ME TO THIS DAY AND HAS CHANGED MY ATTITUDE TO A NUMBER OF THINGS...
"...AND I THINK THAT... WELL, I'M STILL CHANGING, I'M NOT DONE YET.
"BUT IT PUT ME IN A DIFFERENT TIME AND SPACE....IT CHANGED...WELL, IT CHANGED MY SENSE OF THE WORLD AND MY PLACE IN IT."

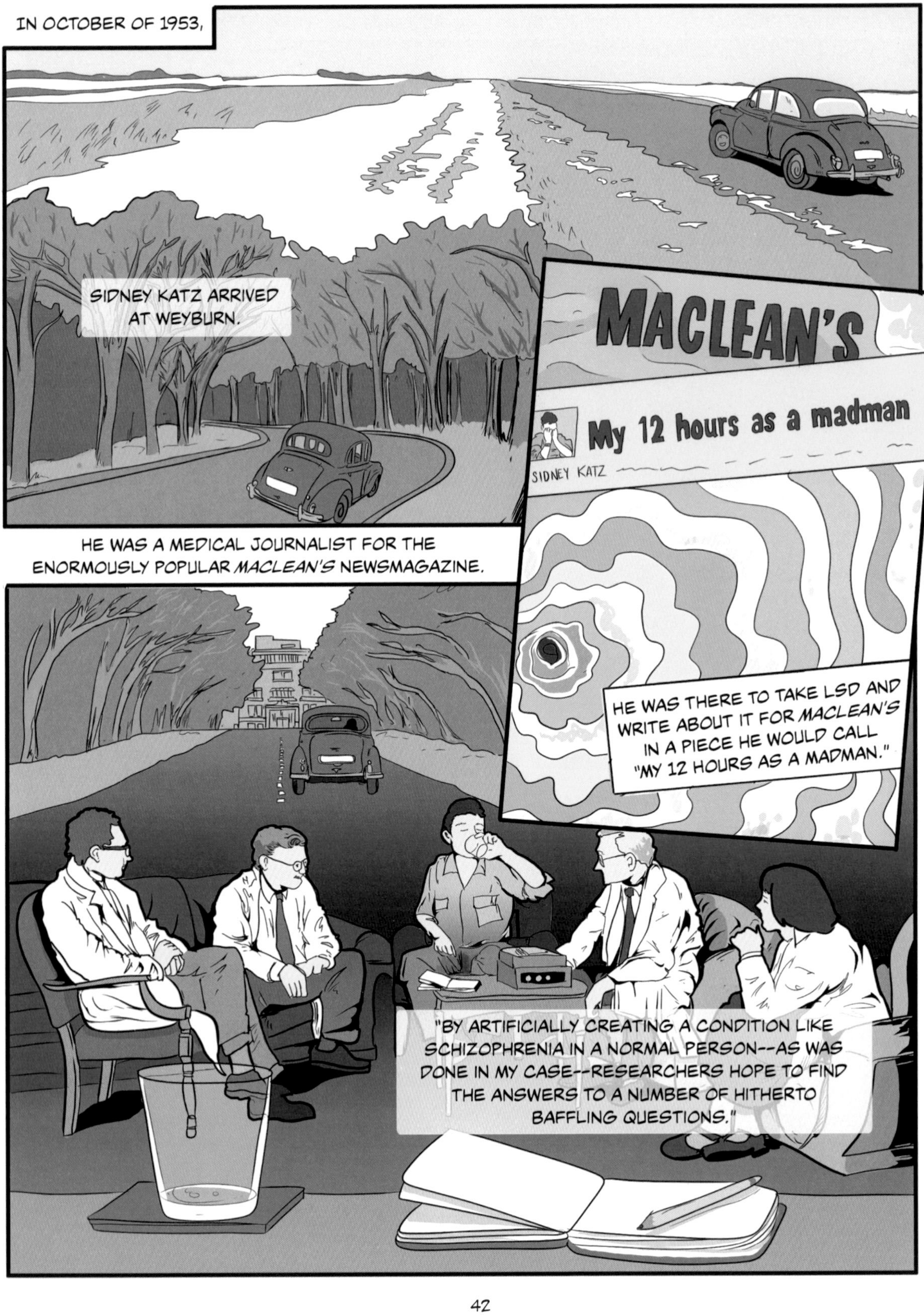
IN OCTOBER OF 1953,
SIDNEY KATZ ARRIVED AT WEYBURN.
MACLEAN'S
My 12 hours as a madman
SIDNEY KATZ
HE WAS A MEDICAL JOURNALIST FOR THE ENORMOUSLY POPULAR *MACLEAN'S* NEWSMAGAZINE.
HE WAS THERE TO TAKE LSD AND WRITE ABOUT IT FOR *MACLEAN'S* IN A PIECE HE WOULD CALL "MY 12 HOURS AS A MADMAN."
"BY ARTIFICIALLY CREATING A CONDITION LIKE SCHIZOPHRENIA IN A NORMAL PERSON--AS WAS DONE IN MY CASE--RESEARCHERS HOPE TO FIND THE ANSWERS TO A NUMBER OF HITHERTO BAFFLING QUESTIONS."

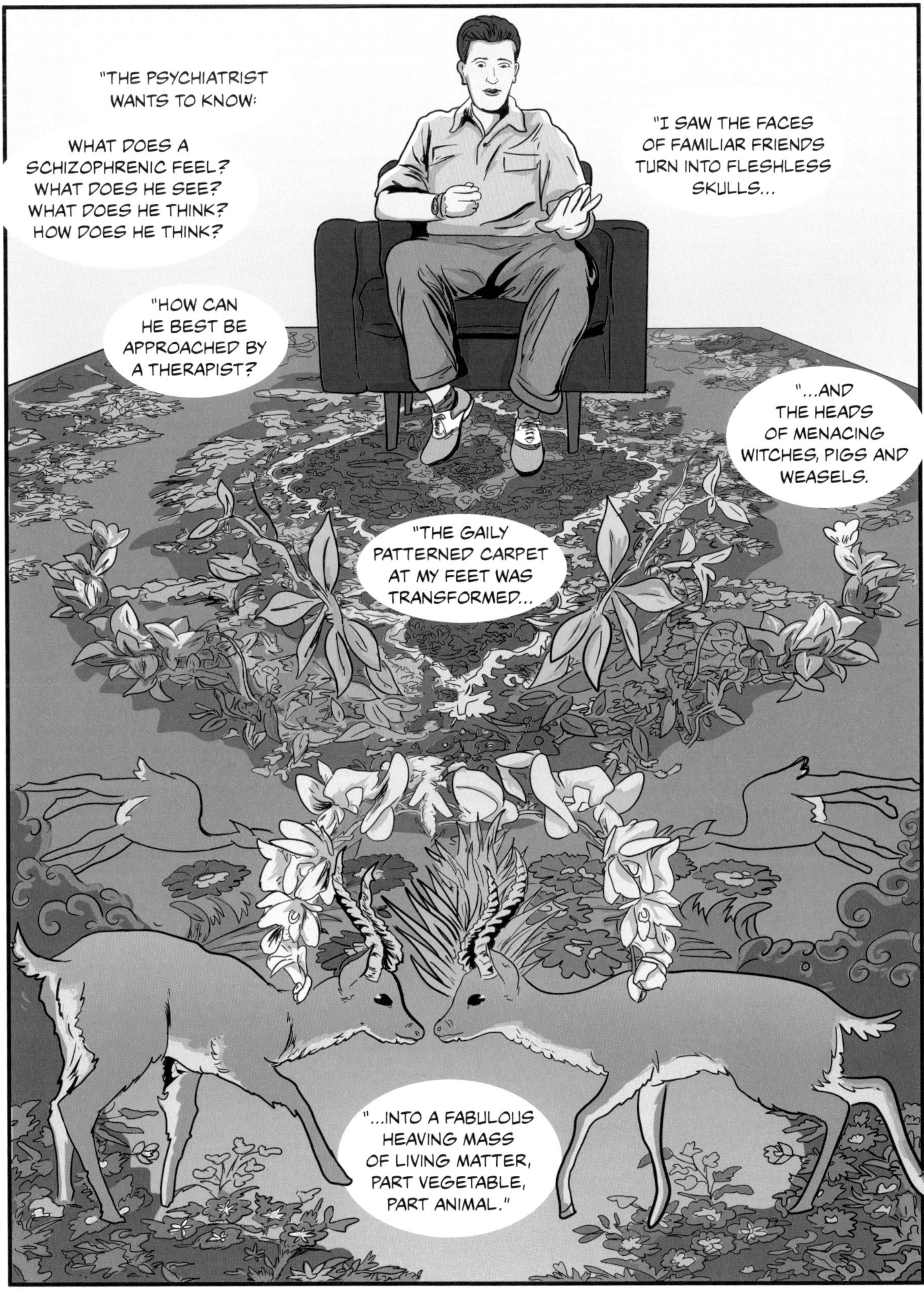
"THE PSYCHIATRIST WANTS TO KNOW:
WHAT DOES A SCHIZOPHRENIC FEEL? WHAT DOES HE SEE? WHAT DOES HE THINK? HOW DOES HE THINK?
"HOW CAN HE BEST BE APPROACHED BY A THERAPIST?
"I SAW THE FACES OF FAMILIAR FRIENDS TURN INTO FLESHLESS SKULLS...
"...AND THE HEADS OF MENACING WITCHES, PIGS AND WEASELS.
"THE GAILY PATTERNED CARPET AT MY FEET WAS TRANSFORMED...
"...INTO A FABULOUS HEAVING MASS OF LIVING MATTER, PART VEGETABLE, PART ANIMAL."

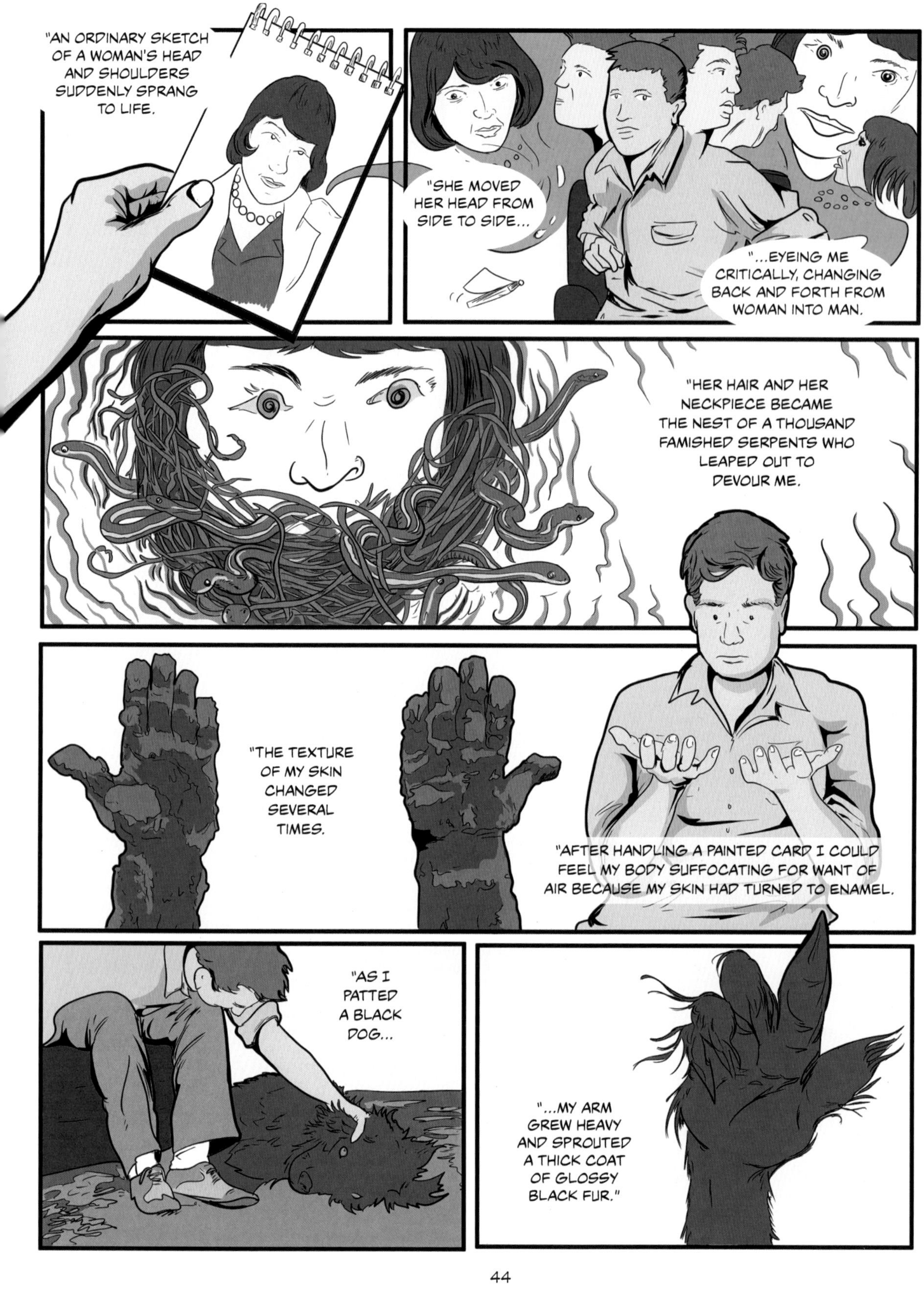

"AN ORDINARY SKETCH OF A WOMAN'S HEAD AND SHOULDERS SUDDENLY SPRANG TO LIFE.
"SHE MOVED HER HEAD FROM SIDE TO SIDE...
"...EYEING ME CRITICALLY, CHANGING BACK AND FORTH FROM WOMAN INTO MAN.
"HER HAIR AND HER NECKPIECE BECAME THE NEST OF A THOUSAND FAMISHED SERPENTS WHO LEAPED OUT TO DEVOUR ME.
"THE TEXTURE OF MY SKIN CHANGED SEVERAL TIMES.
"AFTER HANDLING A PAINTED CARD I COULD FEEL MY BODY SUFFOCATING FOR WANT OF AIR BECAUSE MY SKIN HAD TURNED TO ENAMEL.
"AS I PATTED A BLACK DOG...
"...MY ARM GREW HEAVY AND SPROUTED A THICK COAT OF GLOSSY BLACK FUR."

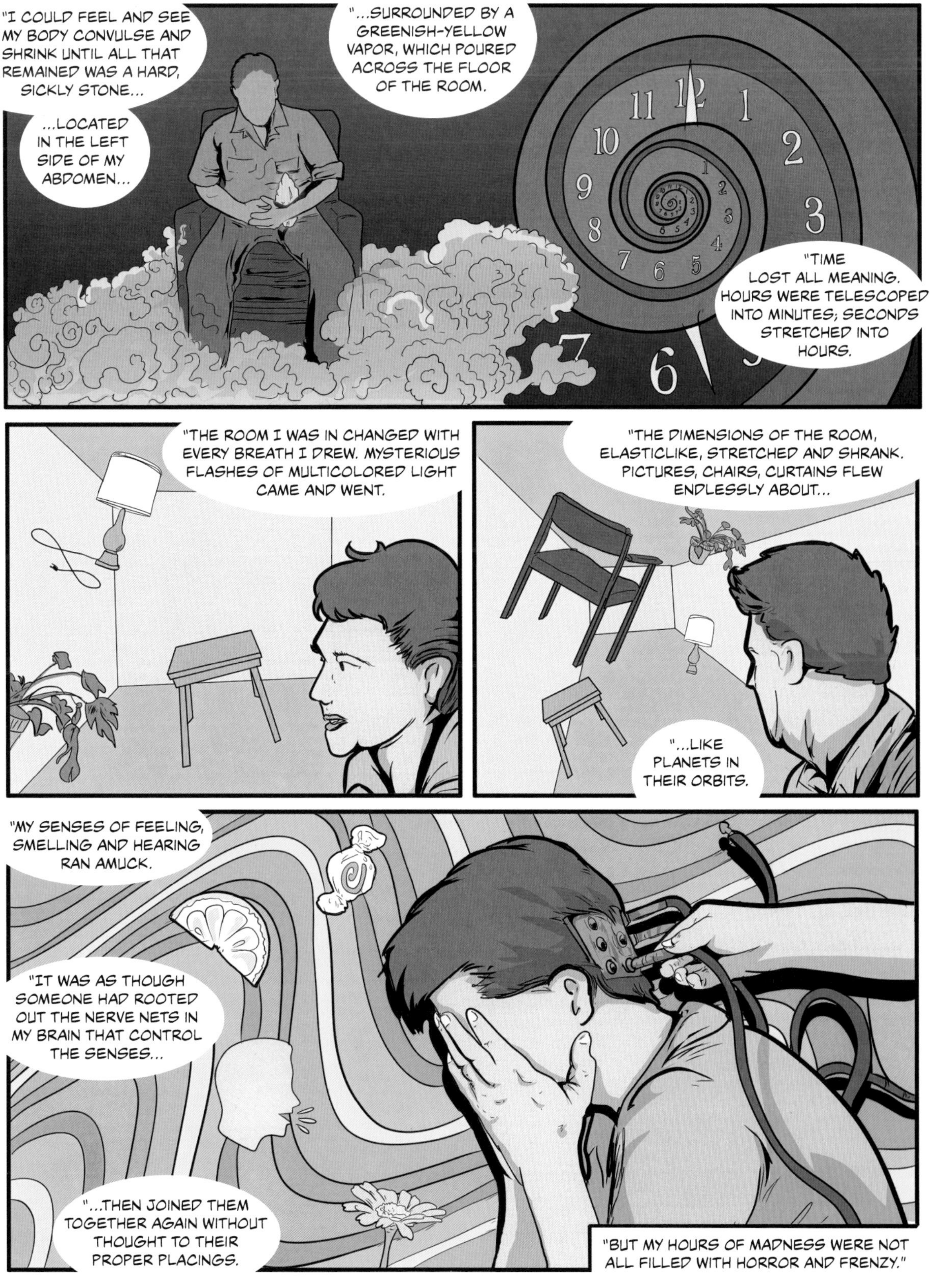
"I COULD FEEL AND SEE MY BODY CONVULSE AND SHRINK UNTIL ALL THAT REMAINED WAS A HARD, SICKLY STONE...
...LOCATED IN THE LEFT SIDE OF MY ABDOMEN...
"...SURROUNDED BY A GREENISH-YELLOW VAPOR, WHICH POURED ACROSS THE FLOOR OF THE ROOM.
"TIME LOST ALL MEANING. HOURS WERE TELESCOPED INTO MINUTES; SECONDS STRETCHED INTO HOURS.
"THE ROOM I WAS IN CHANGED WITH EVERY BREATH I DREW. MYSTERIOUS FLASHES OF MULTICOLORED LIGHT CAME AND WENT.
"THE DIMENSIONS OF THE ROOM, ELASTICLIKE, STRETCHED AND SHRANK. PICTURES, CHAIRS, CURTAINS FLEW ENDLESSLY ABOUT...
"...LIKE PLANETS IN THEIR ORBITS.
"MY SENSES OF FEELING, SMELLING AND HEARING RAN AMUCK.
"IT WAS AS THOUGH SOMEONE HAD ROOTED OUT THE NERVE NETS IN MY BRAIN THAT CONTROL THE SENSES...
"...THEN JOINED THEM TOGETHER AGAIN WITHOUT THOUGHT TO THEIR PROPER PLACINGS.
"BUT MY HOURS OF MADNESS WERE NOT ALL FILLED WITH HORROR AND FRENZY."

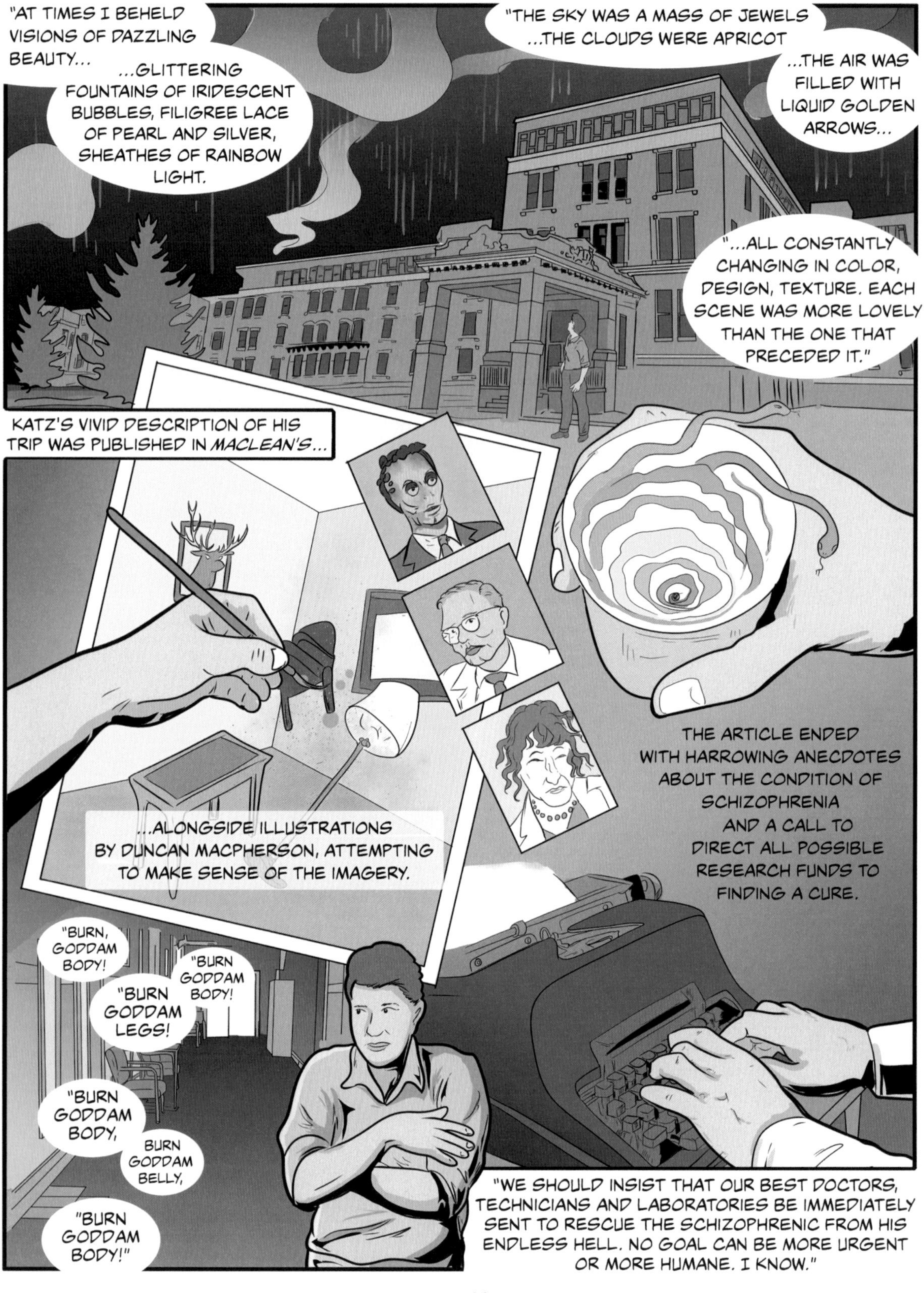
"AT TIMES I BEHELD VISIONS OF DAZZLING BEAUTY...
...GLITTERING FOUNTAINS OF IRIDESCENT BUBBLES, FILIGREE LACE OF PEARL AND SILVER, SHEATHES OF RAINBOW LIGHT.
"THE SKY WAS A MASS OF JEWELS ...THE CLOUDS WERE APRICOT
...THE AIR WAS FILLED WITH LIQUID GOLDEN ARROWS...
"...ALL CONSTANTLY CHANGING IN COLOR, DESIGN, TEXTURE. EACH SCENE WAS MORE LOVELY THAN THE ONE THAT PRECEDED IT."
KATZ'S VIVID DESCRIPTION OF HIS TRIP WAS PUBLISHED IN *MACLEAN'S*...
...ALONGSIDE ILLUSTRATIONS BY DUNCAN MACPHERSON, ATTEMPTING TO MAKE SENSE OF THE IMAGERY.
THE ARTICLE ENDED WITH HARROWING ANECDOTES ABOUT THE CONDITION OF SCHIZOPHRENIA AND A CALL TO DIRECT ALL POSSIBLE RESEARCH FUNDS TO FINDING A CURE.
"BURN, GODDAM BODY!
"BURN GODDAM BODY!
"BURN GODDAM LEGS!
"BURN GODDAM BODY,
BURN GODDAM BELLY,
"BURN GODDAM BODY!"
"WE SHOULD INSIST THAT OUR BEST DOCTORS, TECHNICIANS AND LABORATORIES BE IMMEDIATELY SENT TO RESCUE THE SCHIZOPHRENIC FROM HIS ENDLESS HELL. NO GOAL CAN BE MORE URGENT OR MORE HUMANE. I KNOW."

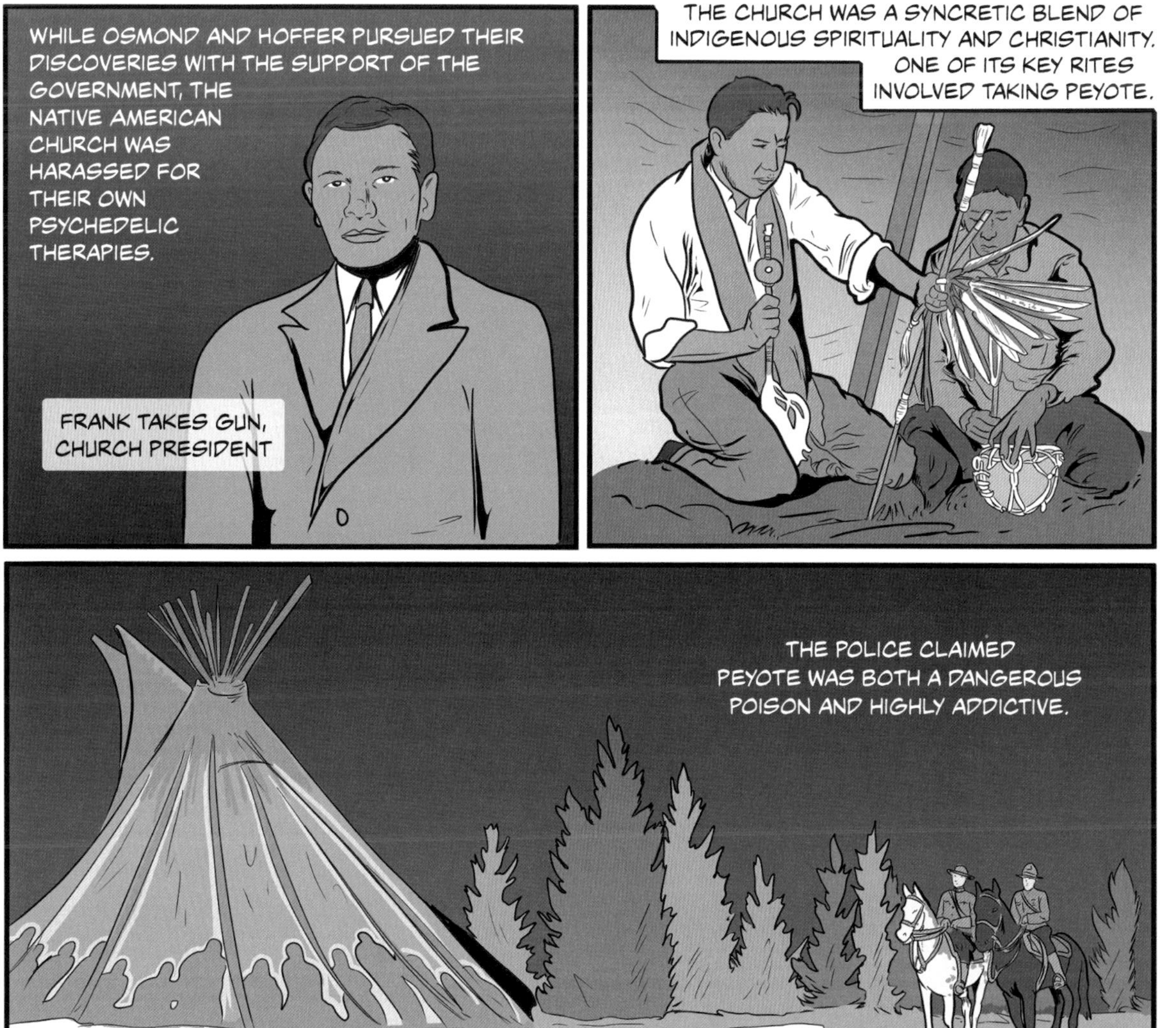
WHILE OSMOND AND HOFFER PURSUED THEIR DISCOVERIES WITH THE SUPPORT OF THE GOVERNMENT, THE NATIVE AMERICAN CHURCH WAS HARASSED FOR THEIR OWN PSYCHEDELIC THERAPIES.
FRANK TAKES GUN, CHURCH PRESIDENT
THE CHURCH WAS A SYNCRETIC BLEND OF INDIGENOUS SPIRITUALITY AND CHRISTIANITY. ONE OF ITS KEY RITES INVOLVED TAKING PEYOTE.
THE POLICE CLAIMED PEYOTE WAS BOTH A DANGEROUS POISON AND HIGHLY ADDICTIVE.
OSMOND WAS SYMPATHETIC TO THE CHURCH'S PLIGHT.
"ANY YOUNG RELIGION USUALLY MANAGES TO OFFEND LONGER ESTABLISHED CHURCHES."

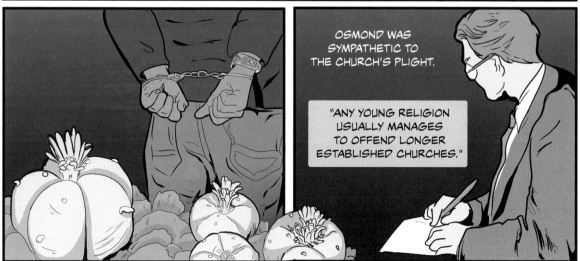

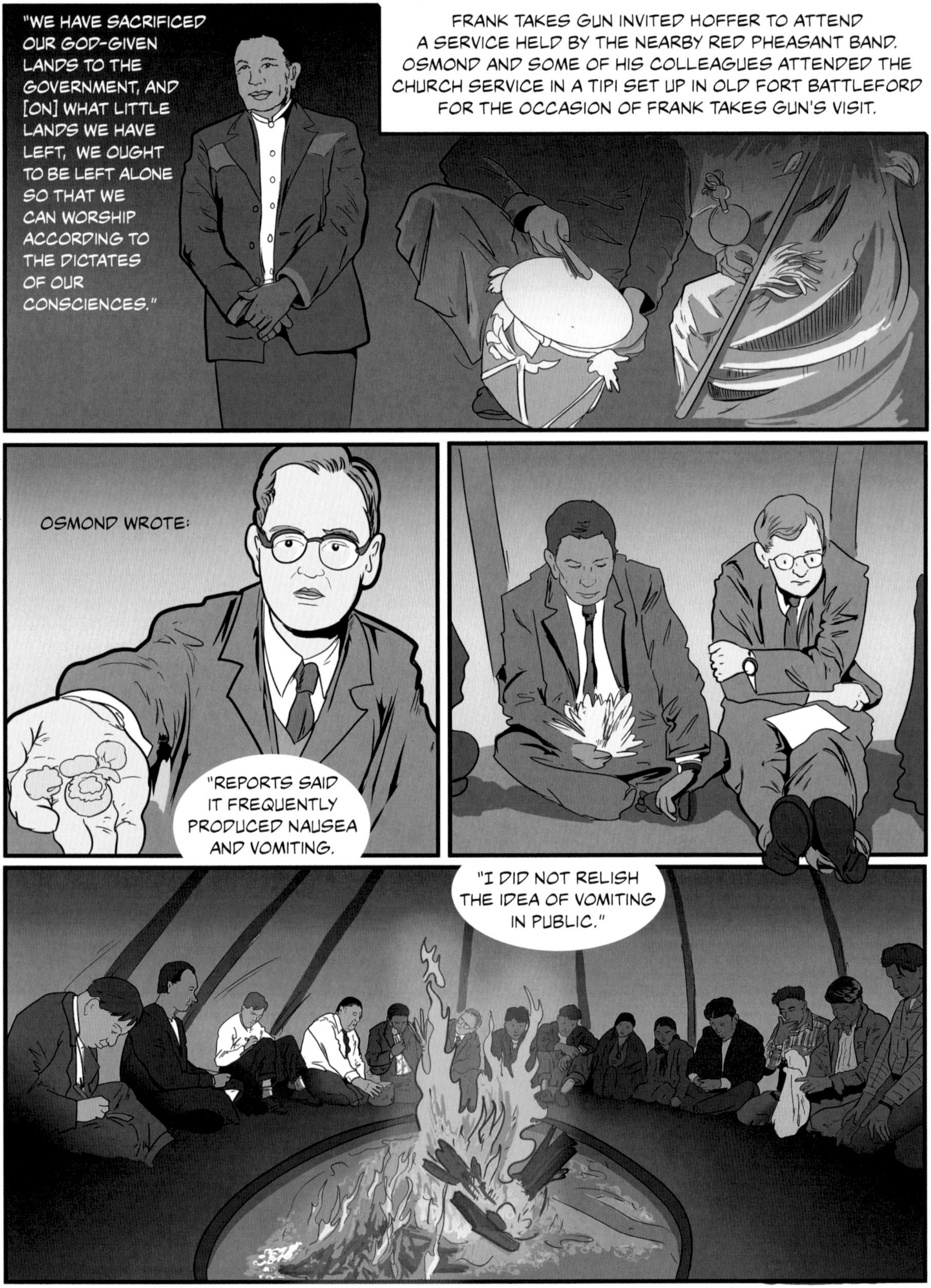
"WE HAVE SACRIFICED OUR GOD-GIVEN LANDS TO THE GOVERNMENT, AND [ON] WHAT LITTLE LANDS WE HAVE LEFT, WE OUGHT TO BE LEFT ALONE SO THAT WE CAN WORSHIP ACCORDING TO THE DICTATES OF OUR CONSCIENCES."
FRANK TAKES GUN INVITED HOFFER TO ATTEND A SERVICE HELD BY THE NEARBY RED PHEASANT BAND. OSMOND AND SOME OF HIS COLLEAGUES ATTENDED THE CHURCH SERVICE IN A TIPI SET UP IN OLD FORT BATTLEFORD FOR THE OCCASION OF FRANK TAKES GUN'S VISIT.
OSMOND WROTE:
"REPORTS SAID IT FREQUENTLY PRODUCED NAUSEA AND VOMITING.
"I DID NOT RELISH THE IDEA OF VOMITING IN PUBLIC."

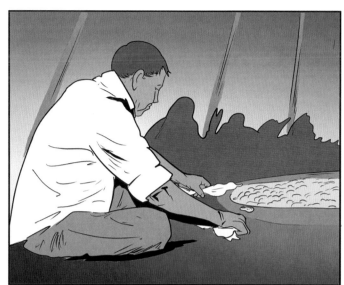

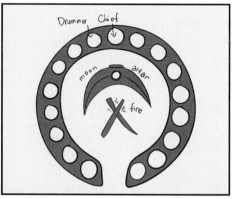

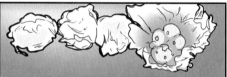

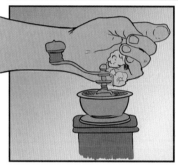

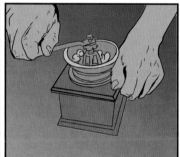

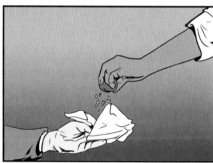

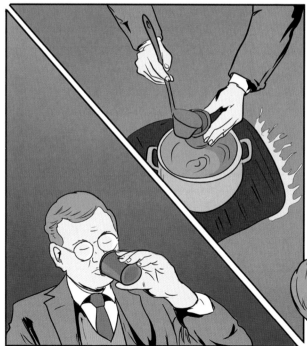

Drummer
Chief
moon
altar
fire
"THE SPARKS SPANGLED IN THE UPPER DARKNESS OF THE TIPI EVERY TIME THE FIRE WAS STOKED."

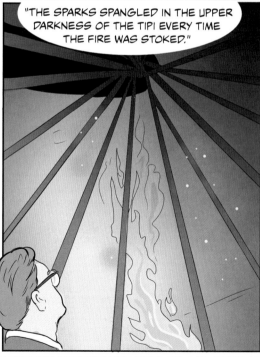

OSMOND LEFT THE EXPERIENCE HUMBLED AND ADMIRING.

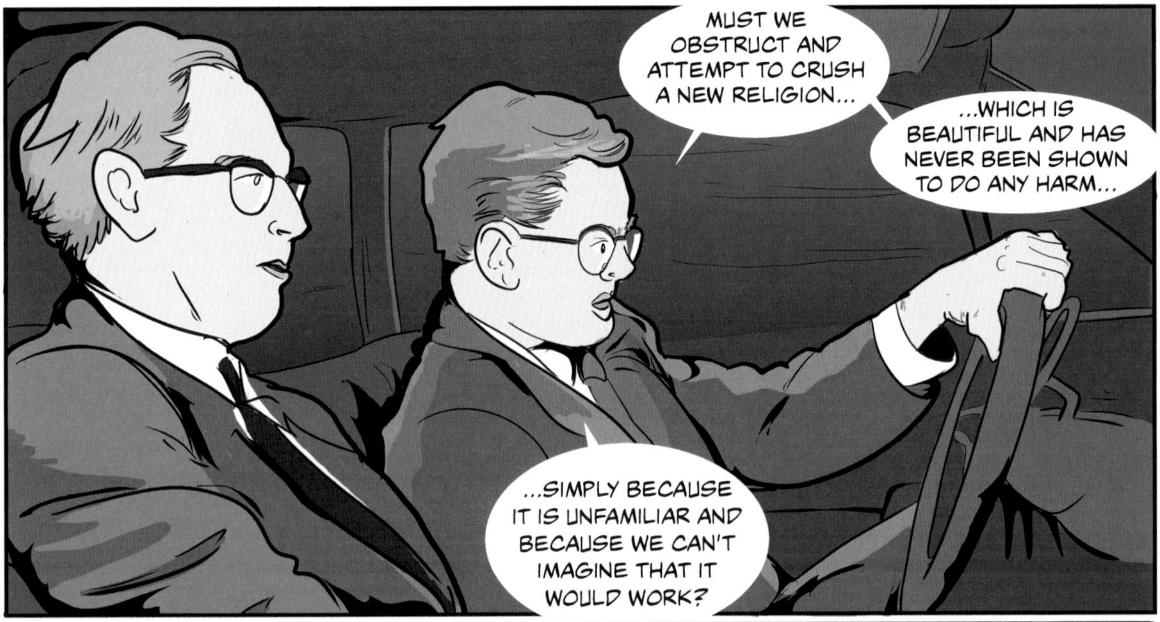
MUST WE OBSTRUCT AND ATTEMPT TO CRUSH A NEW RELIGION...
...WHICH IS BEAUTIFUL AND HAS NEVER BEEN SHOWN TO DO ANY HARM...
...SIMPLY BECAUSE IT IS UNFAMILIAR AND BECAUSE WE CAN'T IMAGINE THAT IT WOULD WORK?

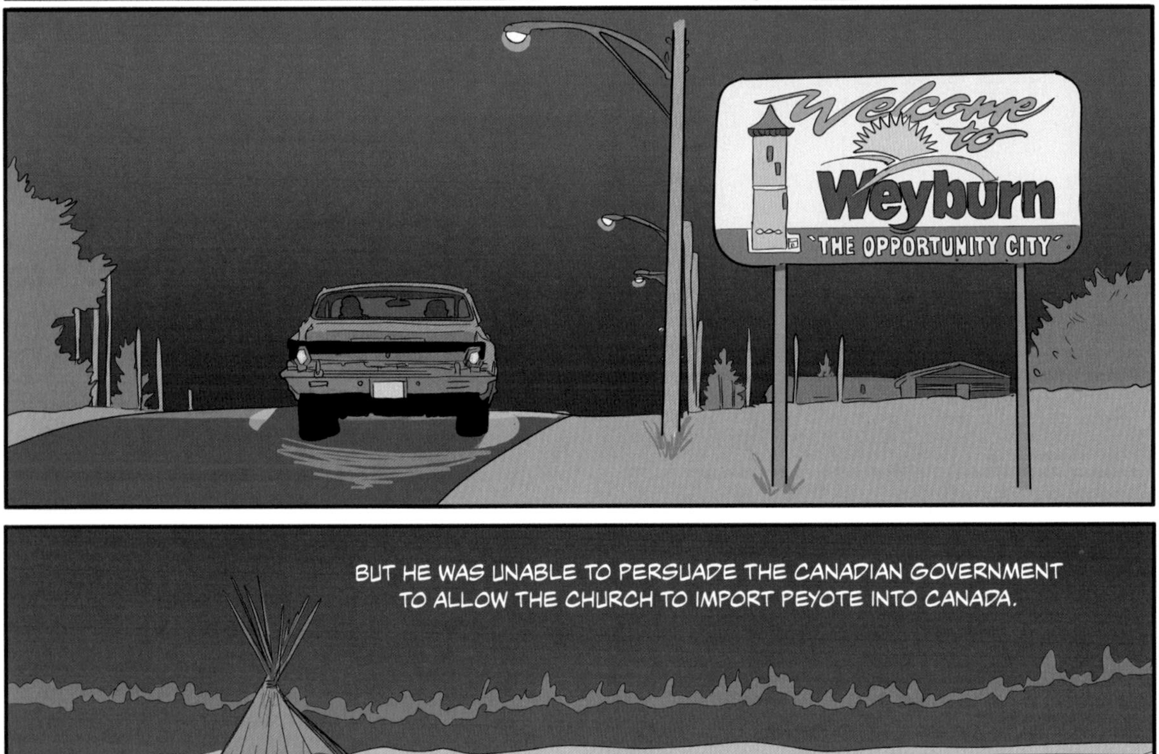
Welcome to
Weyburn
"THE OPPORTUNITY CITY"

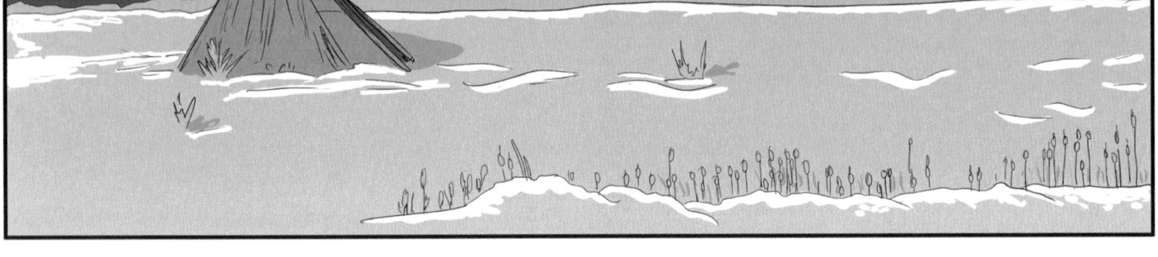
BUT HE WAS UNABLE TO PERSUADE THE CANADIAN GOVERNMENT TO ALLOW THE CHURCH TO IMPORT PEYOTE INTO CANADA.

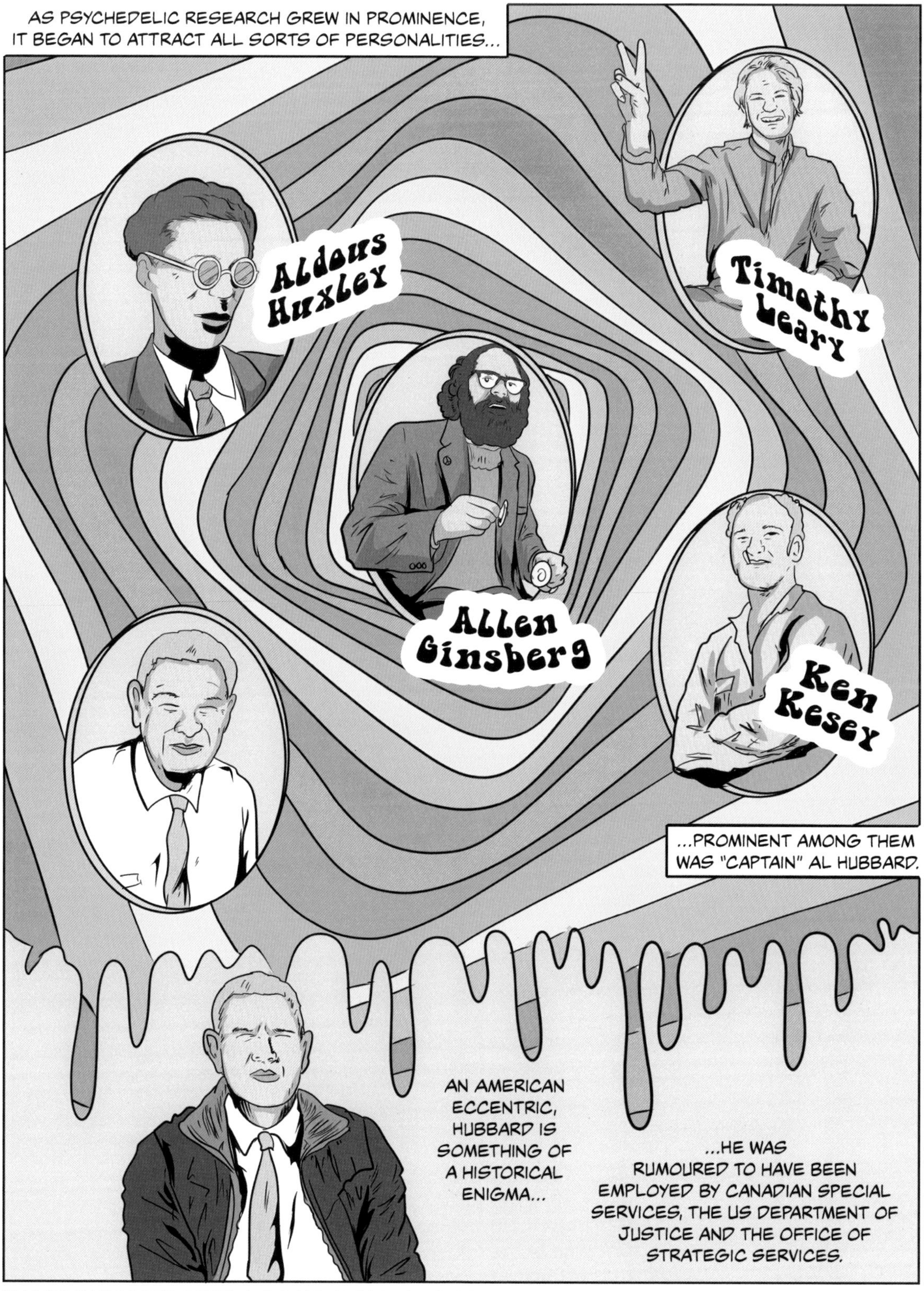
AS PSYCHEDELIC RESEARCH GREW IN PROMINENCE, IT BEGAN TO ATTRACT ALL SORTS OF PERSONALITIES...
Aldous Huxley
Timothy Leary
Allen Ginsberg
Ken Kesey
...PROMINENT AMONG THEM WAS "CAPTAIN" AL HUBBARD.
AN AMERICAN ECCENTRIC, HUBBARD IS SOMETHING OF A HISTORICAL ENIGMA...
...HE WAS RUMOURED TO HAVE BEEN EMPLOYED BY CANADIAN SPECIAL SERVICES, THE US DEPARTMENT OF JUSTICE AND THE OFFICE OF STRATEGIC SERVICES.
WHAT'S KNOWN FOR CERTAIN IS THAT HE PATENTED A "FREE ENERGY" MOTOR--IN OTHER WORDS, A FRAUD--

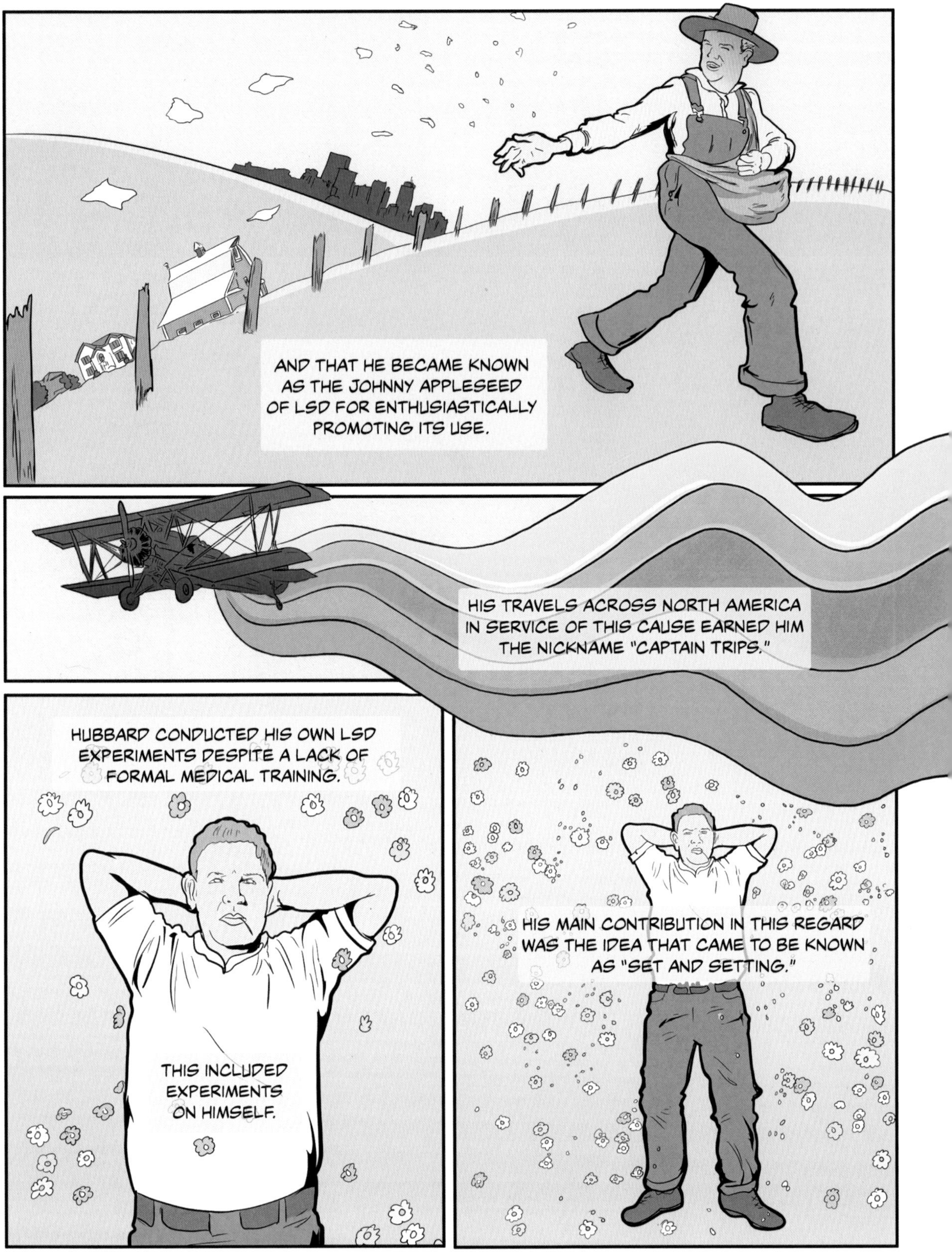
AND THAT HE BECAME KNOWN AS THE JOHNNY APPLESEED OF LSD FOR ENTHUSIASTICALLY PROMOTING ITS USE.
HIS TRAVELS ACROSS NORTH AMERICA IN SERVICE OF THIS CAUSE EARNED HIM THE NICKNAME "CAPTAIN TRIPS."
HUBBARD CONDUCTED HIS OWN LSD EXPERIMENTS DESPITE A LACK OF FORMAL MEDICAL TRAINING.
THIS INCLUDED EXPERIMENTS ON HIMSELF.
HIS MAIN CONTRIBUTION IN THIS REGARD WAS THE IDEA THAT CAME TO BE KNOWN AS "SET AND SETTING."

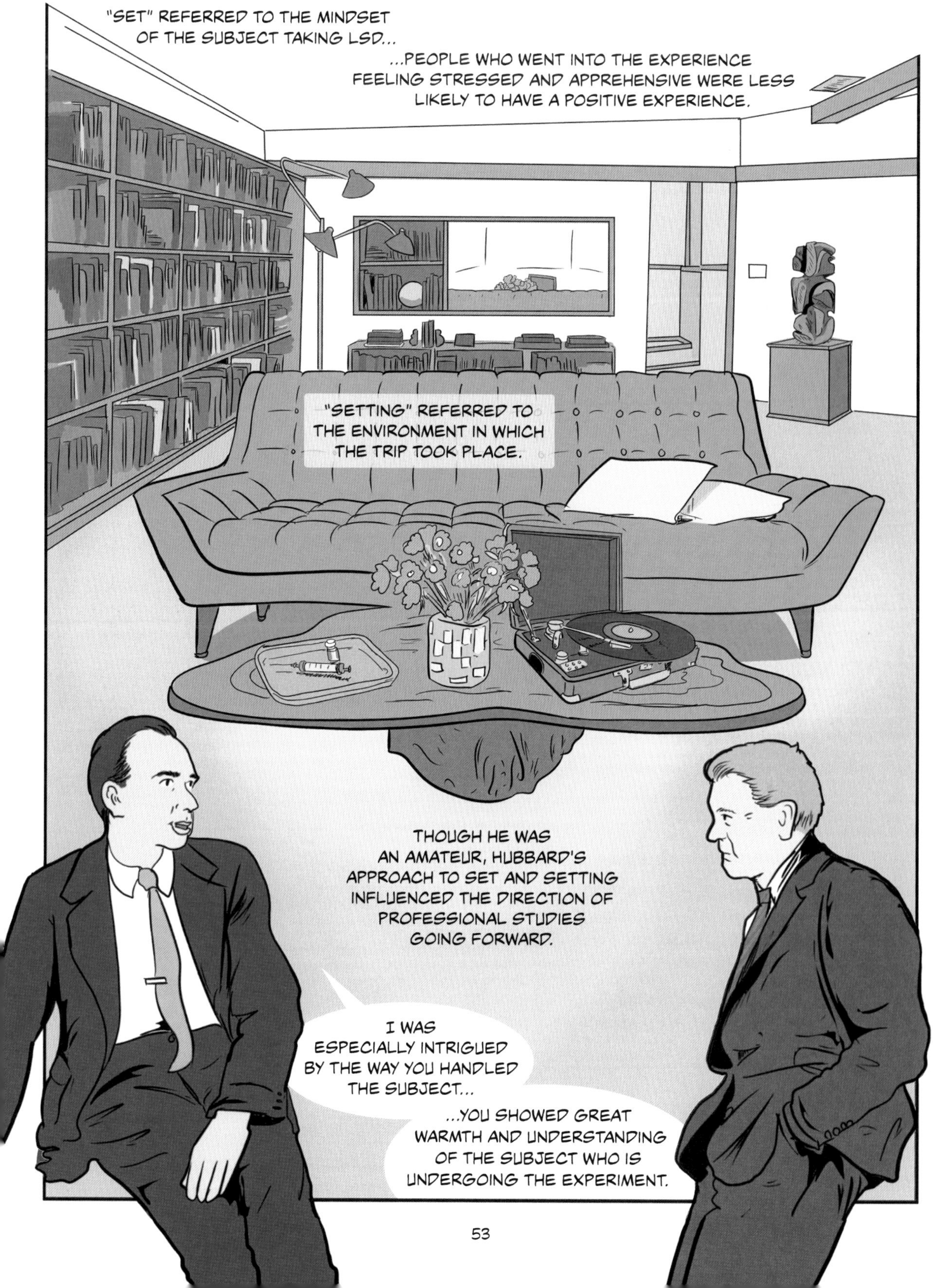
"SET" REFERRED TO THE MINDSET OF THE SUBJECT TAKING LSD...
...PEOPLE WHO WENT INTO THE EXPERIENCE FEELING STRESSED AND APPREHENSIVE WERE LESS LIKELY TO HAVE A POSITIVE EXPERIENCE.
"SETTING" REFERRED TO THE ENVIRONMENT IN WHICH THE TRIP TOOK PLACE.
THOUGH HE WAS AN AMATEUR, HUBBARD'S APPROACH TO SET AND SETTING INFLUENCED THE DIRECTION OF PROFESSIONAL STUDIES GOING FORWARD.
I WAS ESPECIALLY INTRIGUED BY THE WAY YOU HANDLED THE SUBJECT...
...YOU SHOWED GREAT WARMTH AND UNDERSTANDING OF THE SUBJECT WHO IS UNDERGOING THE EXPERIMENT.

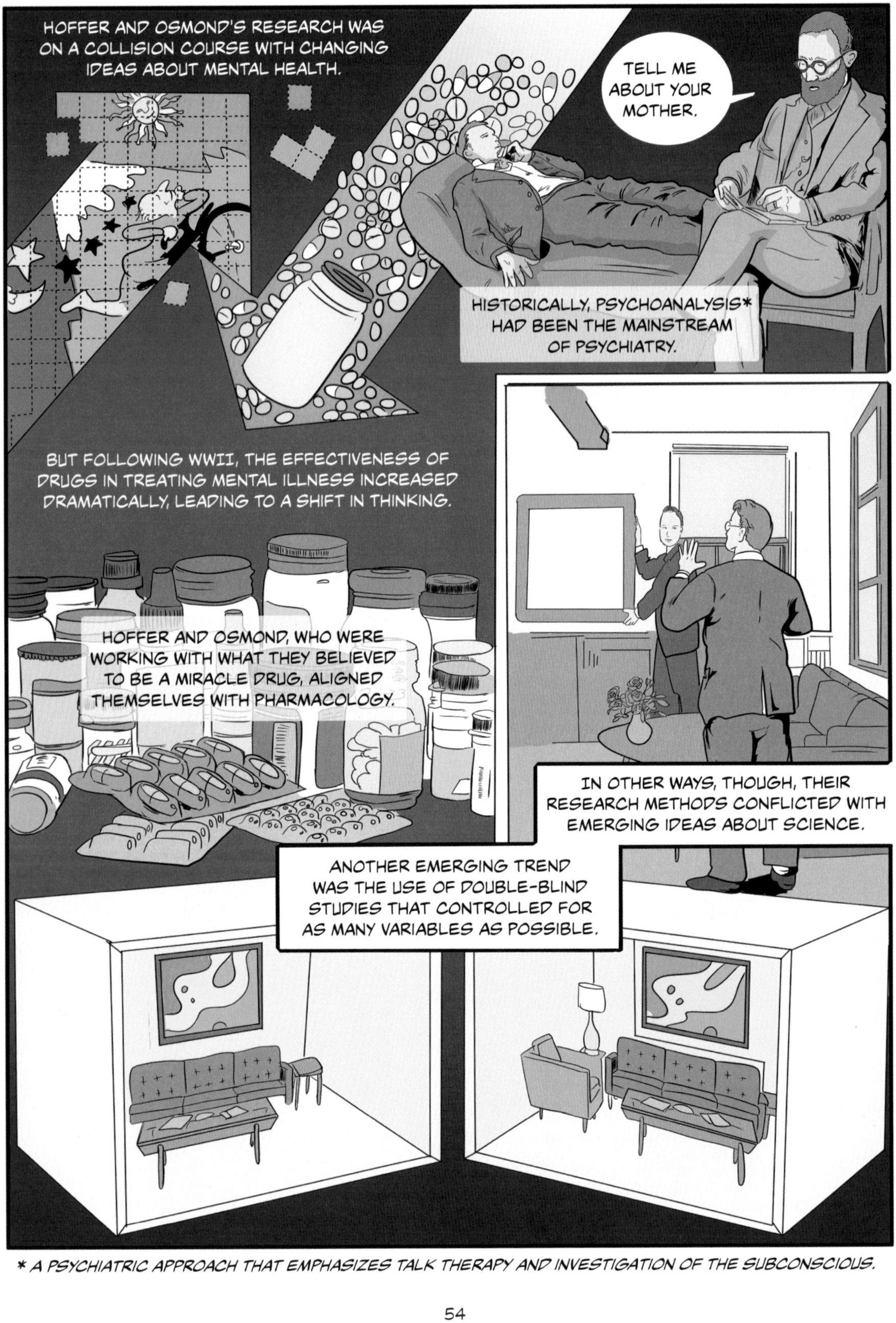
HOFFER AND OSMOND'S RESEARCH WAS ON A COLLISION COURSE WITH CHANGING IDEAS ABOUT MENTAL HEALTH.
TELL ME ABOUT YOUR MOTHER.
HISTORICALLY, PSYCHOANALYSIS* HAD BEEN THE MAINSTREAM OF PSYCHIATRY.
BUT FOLLOWING WWII, THE EFFECTIVENESS OF DRUGS IN TREATING MENTAL ILLNESS INCREASED DRAMATICALLY, LEADING TO A SHIFT IN THINKING.
HOFFER AND OSMOND, WHO WERE WORKING WITH WHAT THEY BELIEVED TO BE A MIRACLE DRUG, ALIGNED THEMSELVES WITH PHARMACOLOGY.
IN OTHER WAYS, THOUGH, THEIR RESEARCH METHODS CONFLICTED WITH EMERGING IDEAS ABOUT SCIENCE.
ANOTHER EMERGING TREND WAS THE USE OF DOUBLE-BLIND STUDIES THAT CONTROLLED FOR AS MANY VARIABLES AS POSSIBLE.

* A PSYCHIATRIC APPROACH THAT EMPHASIZES TALK THERAPY AND INVESTIGATION OF THE SUBCONSCIOUS.

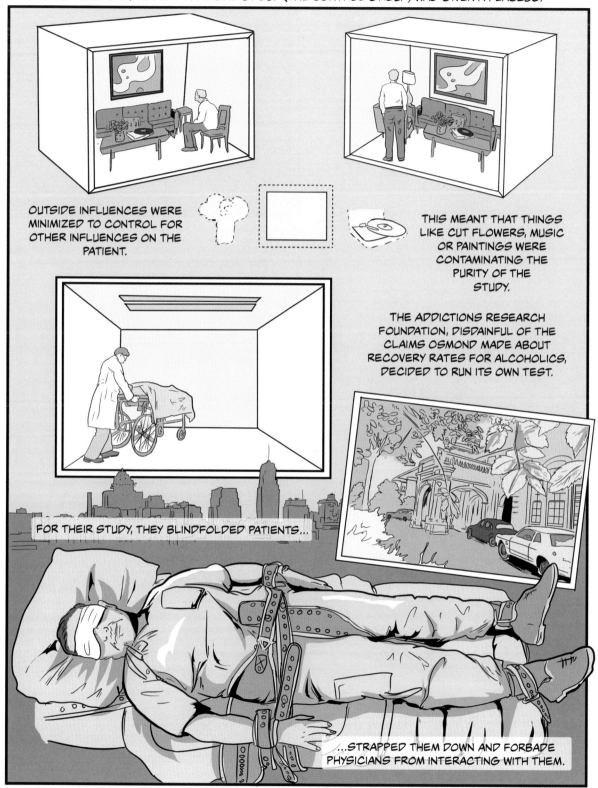

PARTICIPANTS WERE UNAWARE OF THE PURPOSE OF THE STUDY. CONDITIONS WERE AS IDENTICAL AS POSSIBLE, EXCEPT THAT ONE GROUP (THE CONTROL GROUP) WAS GIVEN A PLACEBO.

OUTSIDE INFLUENCES WERE MINIMIZED TO CONTROL FOR OTHER INFLUENCES ON THE PATIENT.

THIS MEANT THAT THINGS LIKE CUT FLOWERS, MUSIC OR PAINTINGS WERE CONTAMINATING THE PURITY OF THE STUDY.

THE ADDICTIONS RESEARCH FOUNDATION, DISDAINFUL OF THE CLAIMS OSMOND MADE ABOUT RECOVERY RATES FOR ALCOHOLICS, DECIDED TO RUN ITS OWN TEST.

FOR THEIR STUDY, THEY BLINDFOLDED PATIENTS...

...STRAPPED THEM DOWN AND FORBADE PHYSICIANS FROM INTERACTING WITH THEM.

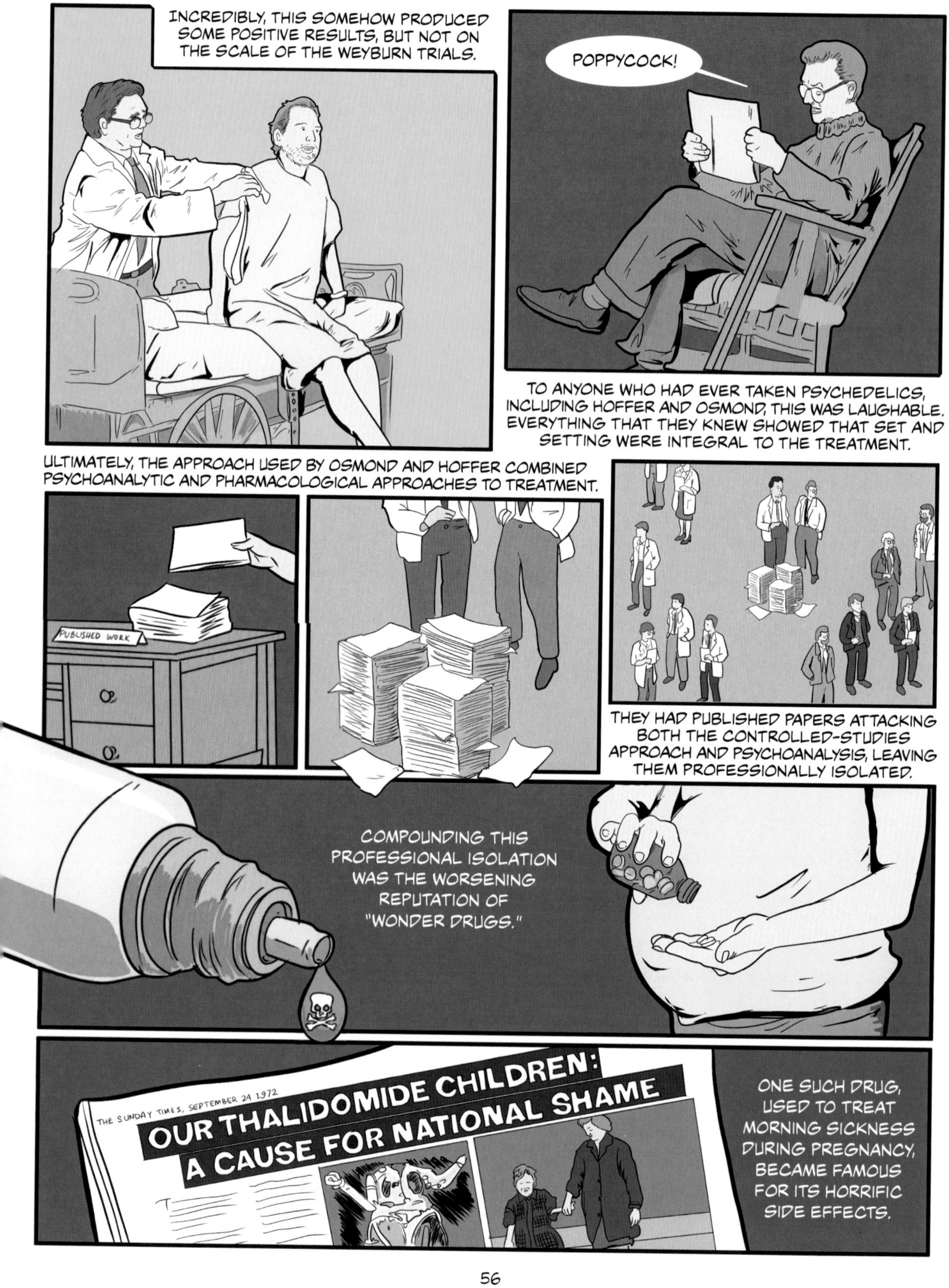
INCREDIBLY, THIS SOMEHOW PRODUCED SOME POSITIVE RESULTS, BUT NOT ON THE SCALE OF THE WEYBURN TRIALS.
POPPYCOCK!
TO ANYONE WHO HAD EVER TAKEN PSYCHEDELICS, INCLUDING HOFFER AND OSMOND, THIS WAS LAUGHABLE. EVERYTHING THAT THEY KNEW SHOWED THAT SET AND SETTING WERE INTEGRAL TO THE TREATMENT.
ULTIMATELY, THE APPROACH USED BY OSMOND AND HOFFER COMBINED PSYCHOANALYTIC AND PHARMACOLOGICAL APPROACHES TO TREATMENT.
PUBLISHED WORK
THEY HAD PUBLISHED PAPERS ATTACKING BOTH THE CONTROLLED-STUDIES APPROACH AND PSYCHOANALYSIS, LEAVING THEM PROFESSIONALLY ISOLATED.
COMPOUNDING THIS PROFESSIONAL ISOLATION WAS THE WORSENING REPUTATION OF "WONDER DRUGS."
THE SUNDAY TIMES, SEPTEMBER 24 1972
OUR THALIDOMIDE CHILDREN: A CAUSE FOR NATIONAL SHAME
ONE SUCH DRUG, USED TO TREAT MORNING SICKNESS DURING PREGNANCY, BECAME FAMOUS FOR ITS HORRIFIC SIDE EFFECTS.

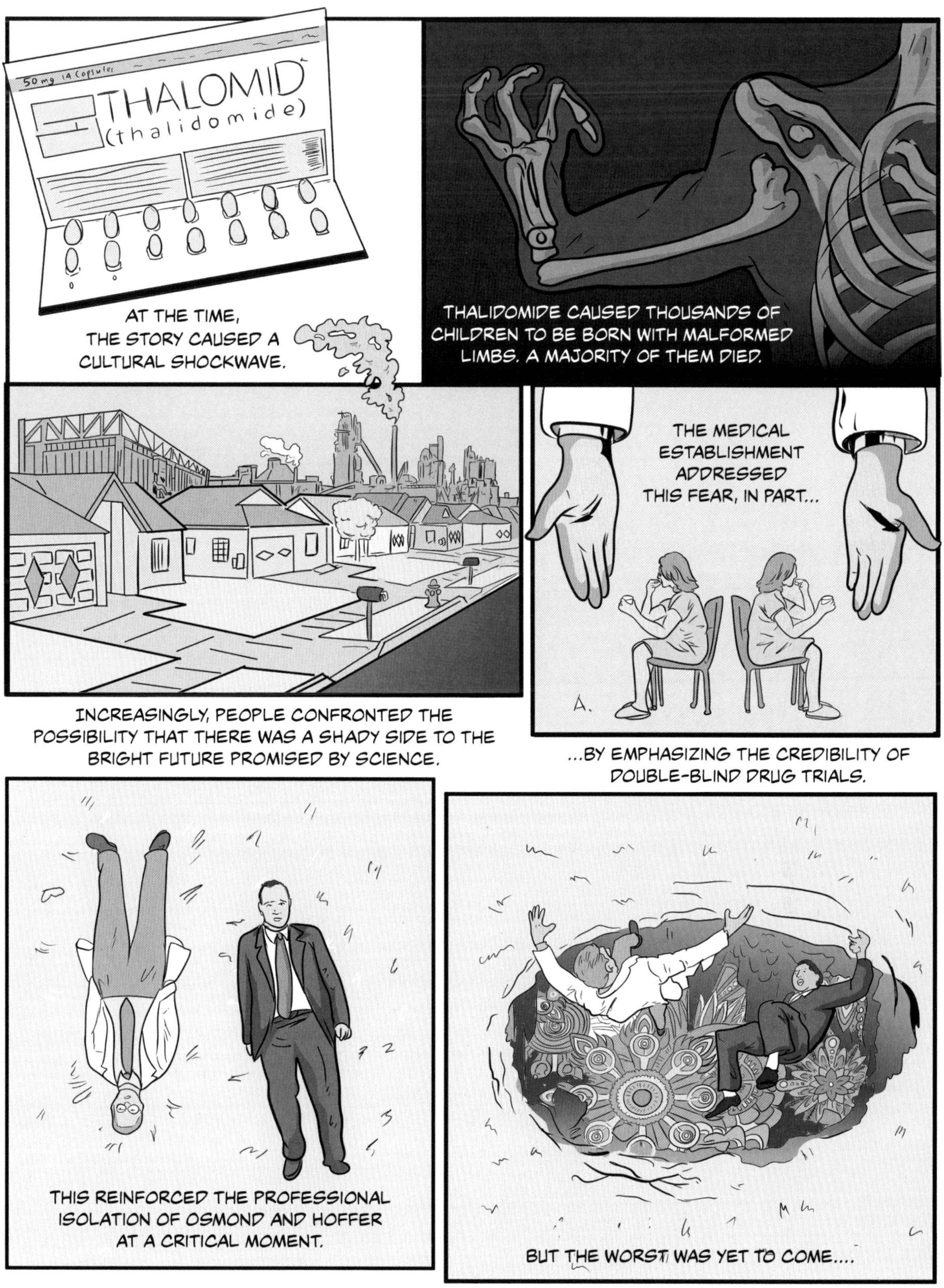
50 mg 14 Capsules
THALOMID
(thalidomide)
AT THE TIME, THE STORY CAUSED A CULTURAL SHOCKWAVE.
THALIDOMIDE CAUSED THOUSANDS OF CHILDREN TO BE BORN WITH MALFORMED LIMBS. A MAJORITY OF THEM DIED.
INCREASINGLY, PEOPLE CONFRONTED THE POSSIBILITY THAT THERE WAS A SHADY SIDE TO THE BRIGHT FUTURE PROMISED BY SCIENCE.
THE MEDICAL ESTABLISHMENT ADDRESSED THIS FEAR, IN PART...
A.
...BY EMPHASIZING THE CREDIBILITY OF DOUBLE-BLIND DRUG TRIALS.
THIS REINFORCED THE PROFESSIONAL ISOLATION OF OSMOND AND HOFFER AT A CRITICAL MOMENT.
BUT THE WORST WAS YET TO COME....

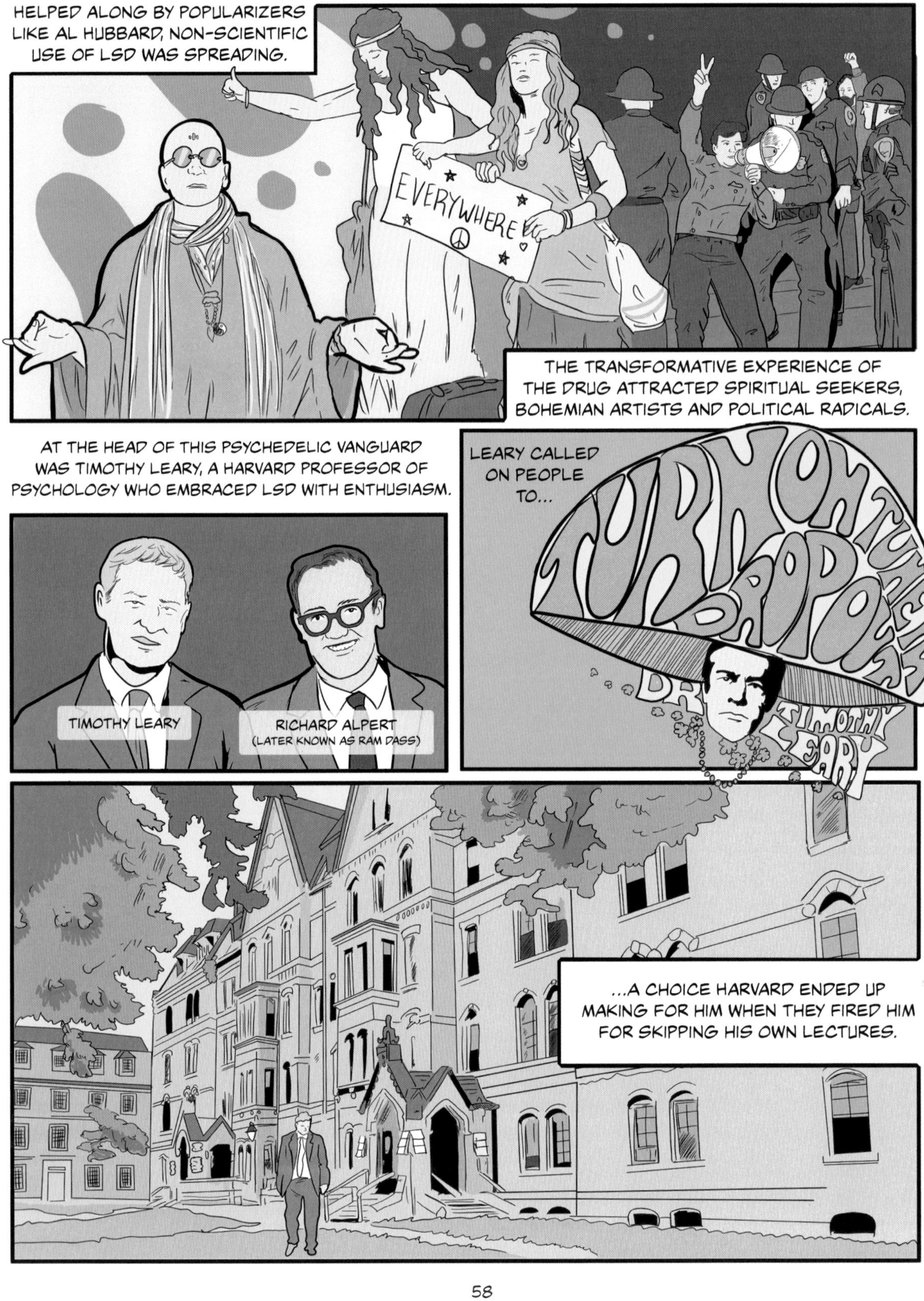
HELPED ALONG BY POPULARIZERS LIKE AL HUBBARD, NON-SCIENTIFIC USE OF LSD WAS SPREADING.
EVERYWHERE
THE TRANSFORMATIVE EXPERIENCE OF THE DRUG ATTRACTED SPIRITUAL SEEKERS, BOHEMIAN ARTISTS AND POLITICAL RADICALS.
AT THE HEAD OF THIS PSYCHEDELIC VANGUARD WAS TIMOTHY LEARY, A HARVARD PROFESSOR OF PSYCHOLOGY WHO EMBRACED LSD WITH ENTHUSIASM.
TIMOTHY LEARY
RICHARD ALPERT (LATER KNOWN AS RAM DASS)
LEARY CALLED ON PEOPLE TO...
TURN ON TUNE IN DROP OUT
TIMOTHY LEARY
...A CHOICE HARVARD ENDED UP MAKING FOR HIM WHEN THEY FIRED HIM FOR SKIPPING HIS OWN LECTURES.

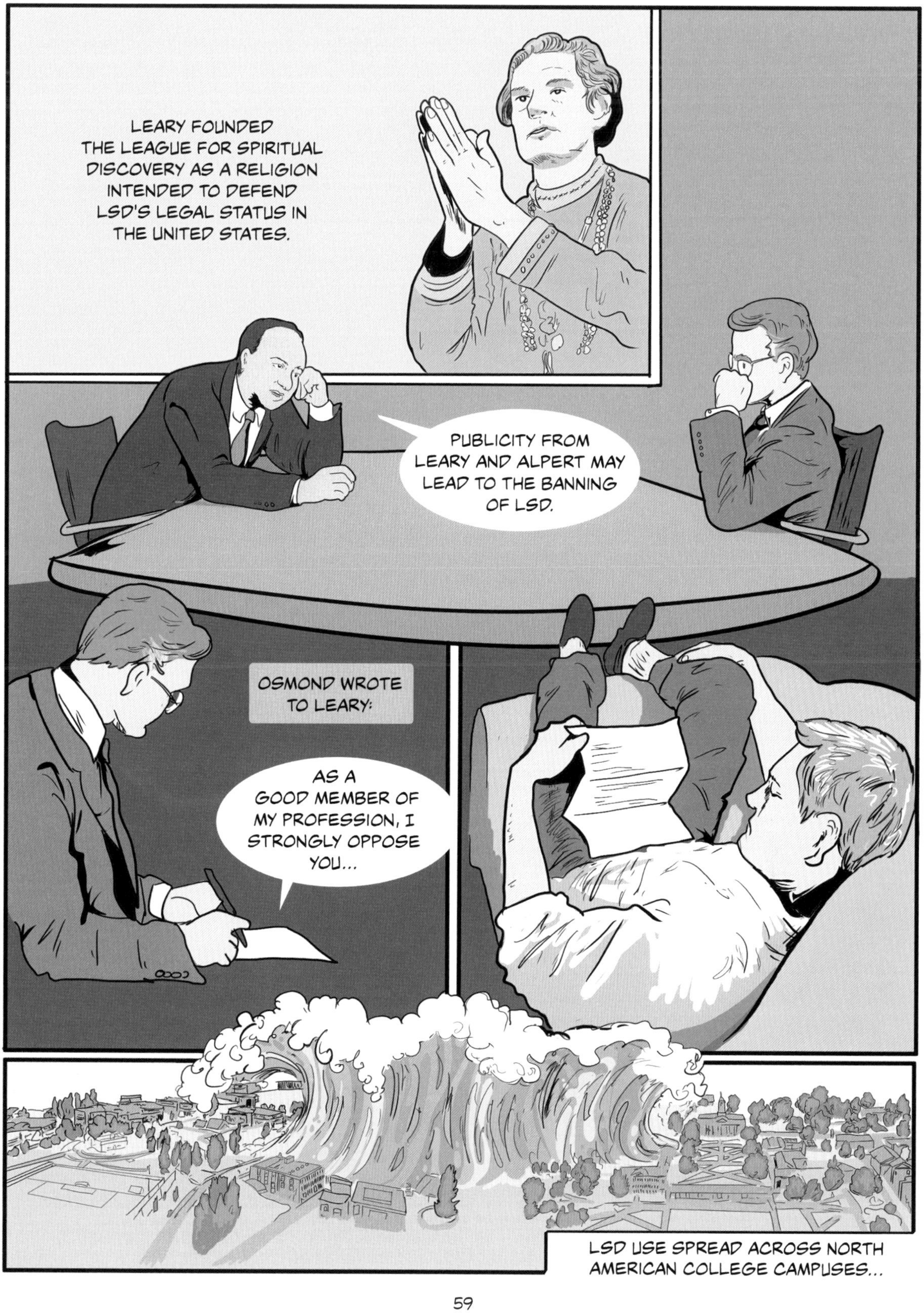
LEARY FOUNDED THE LEAGUE FOR SPIRITUAL DISCOVERY AS A RELIGION INTENDED TO DEFEND LSD'S LEGAL STATUS IN THE UNITED STATES.
PUBLICITY FROM LEARY AND ALPERT MAY LEAD TO THE BANNING OF LSD.
OSMOND WROTE TO LEARY:
AS A GOOD MEMBER OF MY PROFESSION, I STRONGLY OPPOSE YOU...
LSD USE SPREAD ACROSS NORTH AMERICAN COLLEGE CAMPUSES...

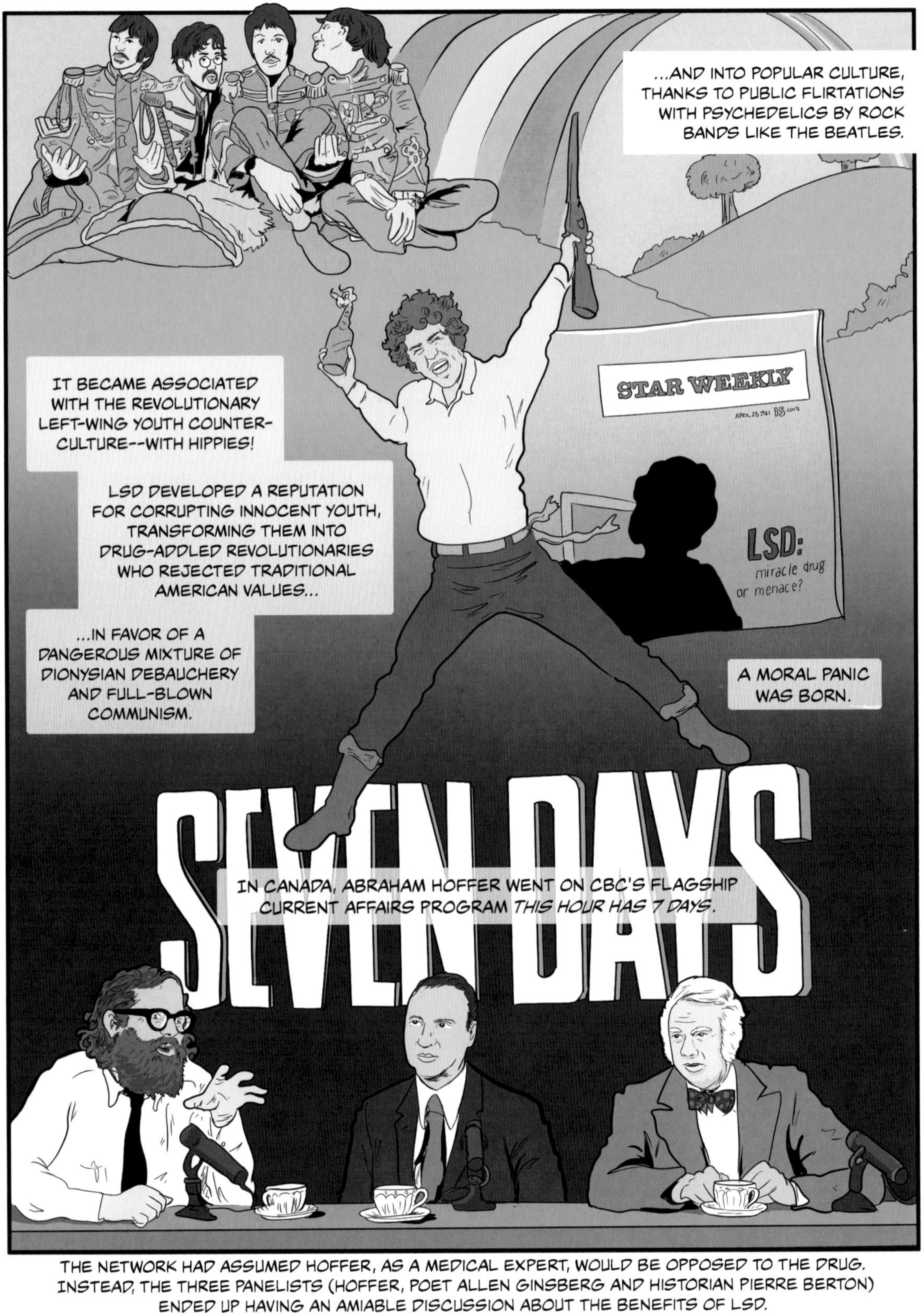
...AND INTO POPULAR CULTURE, THANKS TO PUBLIC FLIRTATIONS WITH PSYCHEDELICS BY ROCK BANDS LIKE THE BEATLES.
IT BECAME ASSOCIATED WITH THE REVOLUTIONARY LEFT-WING YOUTH COUNTER-CULTURE--WITH HIPPIES!
STAR WEEKLY
LSD DEVELOPED A REPUTATION FOR CORRUPTING INNOCENT YOUTH, TRANSFORMING THEM INTO DRUG-ADDLED REVOLUTIONARIES WHO REJECTED TRADITIONAL AMERICAN VALUES...
LSD: miracle drug or menace?
...IN FAVOR OF A DANGEROUS MIXTURE OF DIONYSIAN DEBAUCHERY AND FULL-BLOWN COMMUNISM.
A MORAL PANIC WAS BORN.
SEVEN DAYS
IN CANADA, ABRAHAM HOFFER WENT ON CBC'S FLAGSHIP CURRENT AFFAIRS PROGRAM *THIS HOUR HAS 7 DAYS*.

THE NETWORK HAD ASSUMED HOFFER, AS A MEDICAL EXPERT, WOULD BE OPPOSED TO THE DRUG. INSTEAD, THE THREE PANELISTS (HOFFER, POET ALLEN GINSBERG AND HISTORIAN PIERRE BERTON) ENDED UP HAVING AN AMIABLE DISCUSSION ABOUT THE BENEFITS OF LSD.

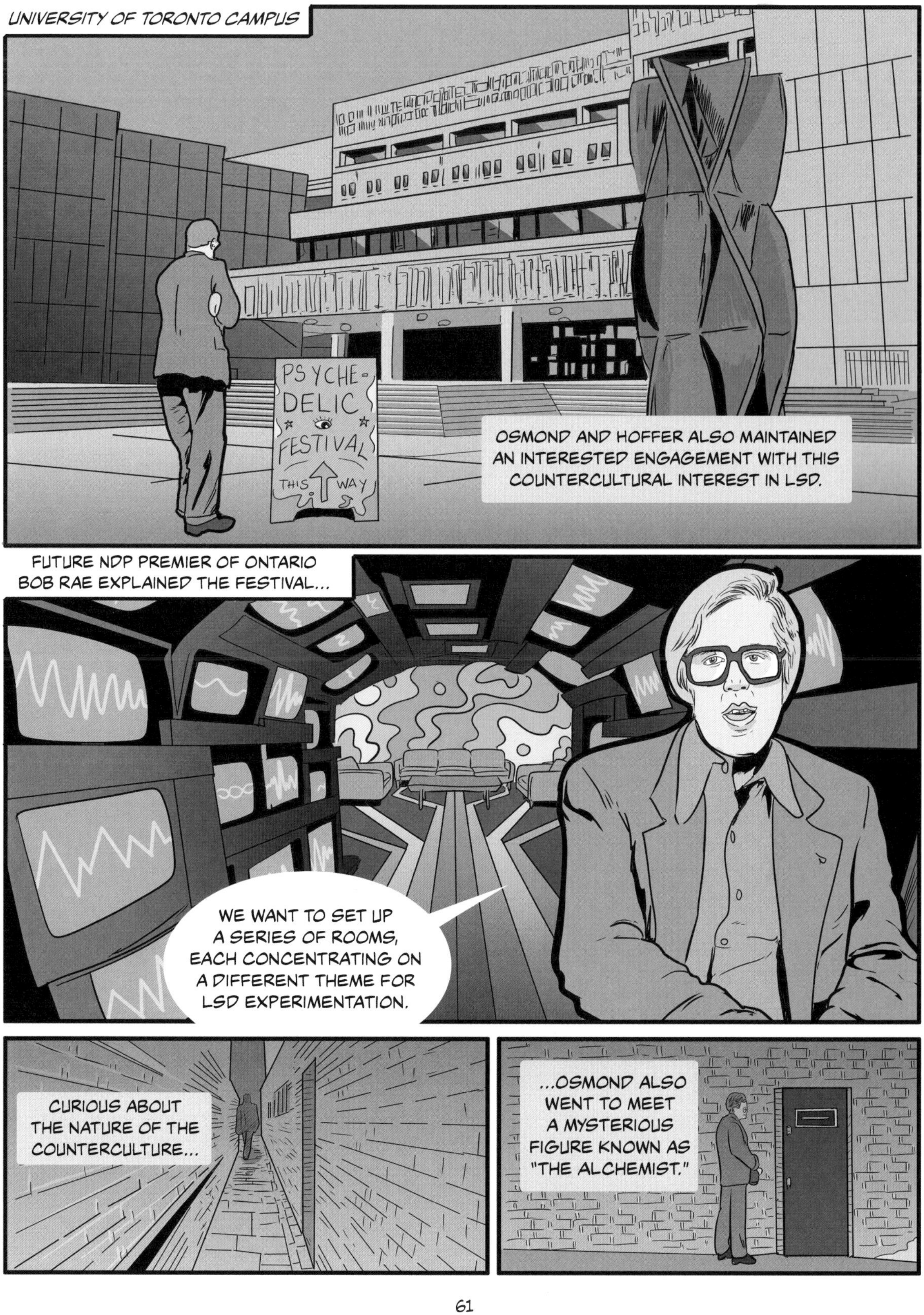
UNIVERSITY OF TORONTO CAMPUS
PSYCHE-DELIC FESTIVAL THIS WAY
OSMOND AND HOFFER ALSO MAINTAINED AN INTERESTED ENGAGEMENT WITH THIS COUNTERCULTURAL INTEREST IN LSD.
FUTURE NDP PREMIER OF ONTARIO BOB RAE EXPLAINED THE FESTIVAL...
WE WANT TO SET UP A SERIES OF ROOMS, EACH CONCENTRATING ON A DIFFERENT THEME FOR LSD EXPERIMENTATION.
CURIOUS ABOUT THE NATURE OF THE COUNTERCULTURE...
...OSMOND ALSO WENT TO MEET A MYSTERIOUS FIGURE KNOWN AS "THE ALCHEMIST."

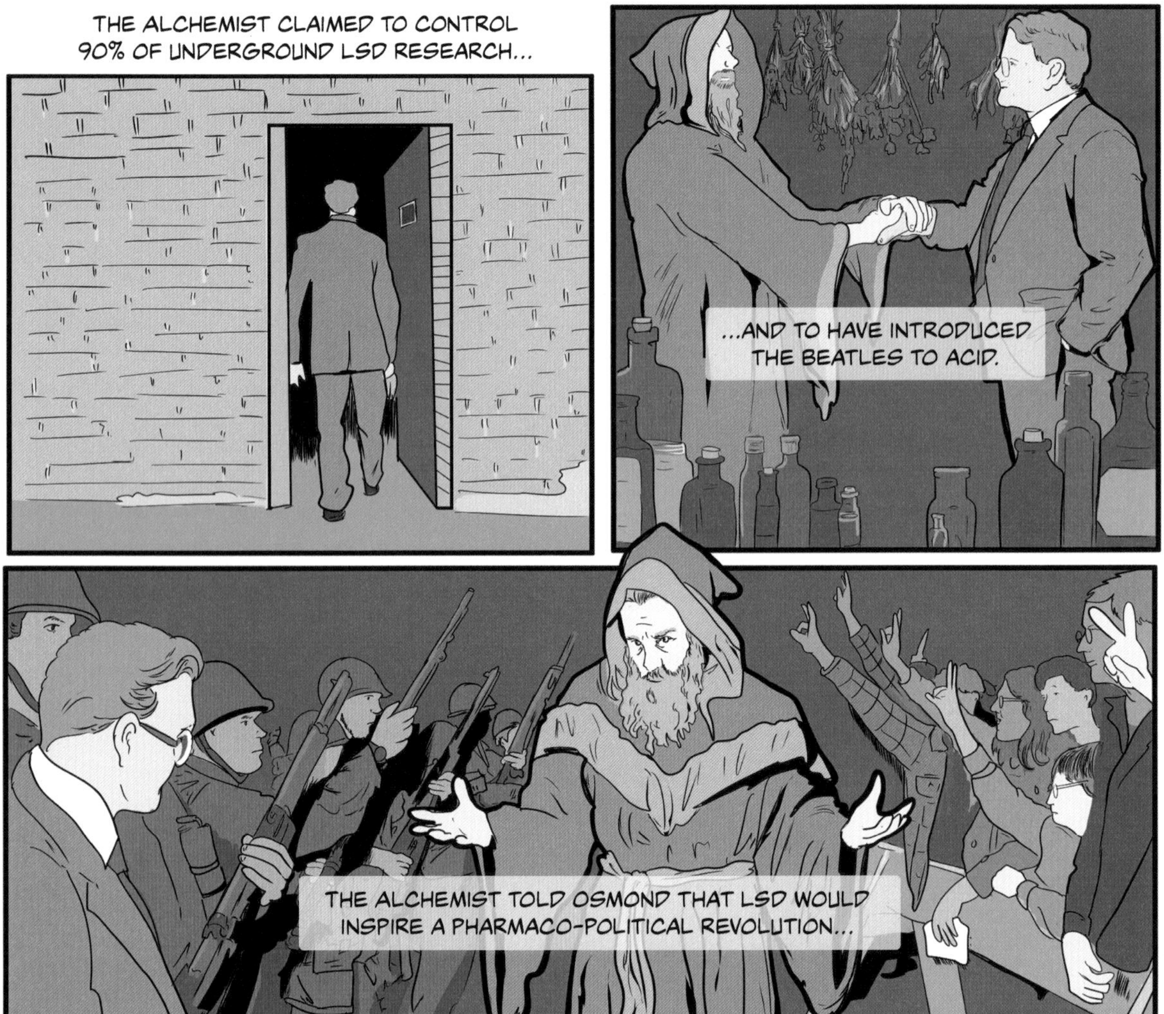
THE ALCHEMIST CLAIMED TO CONTROL 90% OF UNDERGROUND LSD RESEARCH...
...AND TO HAVE INTRODUCED THE BEATLES TO ACID.
THE ALCHEMIST TOLD OSMOND THAT LSD WOULD INSPIRE A PHARMACO-POLITICAL REVOLUTION...
...THAT WOULD SAVE MANKIND FROM THE DANGERS OF THE BOMB...
...AND THE MECHANISTIC, INHUMAN CONFORMITY OF MODERN LIFE.

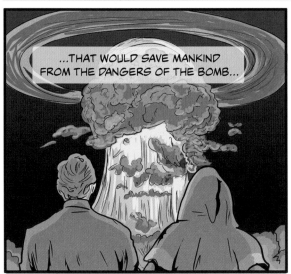

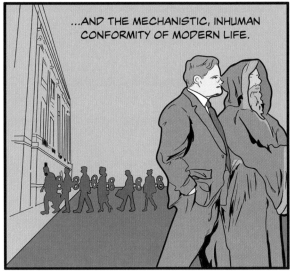

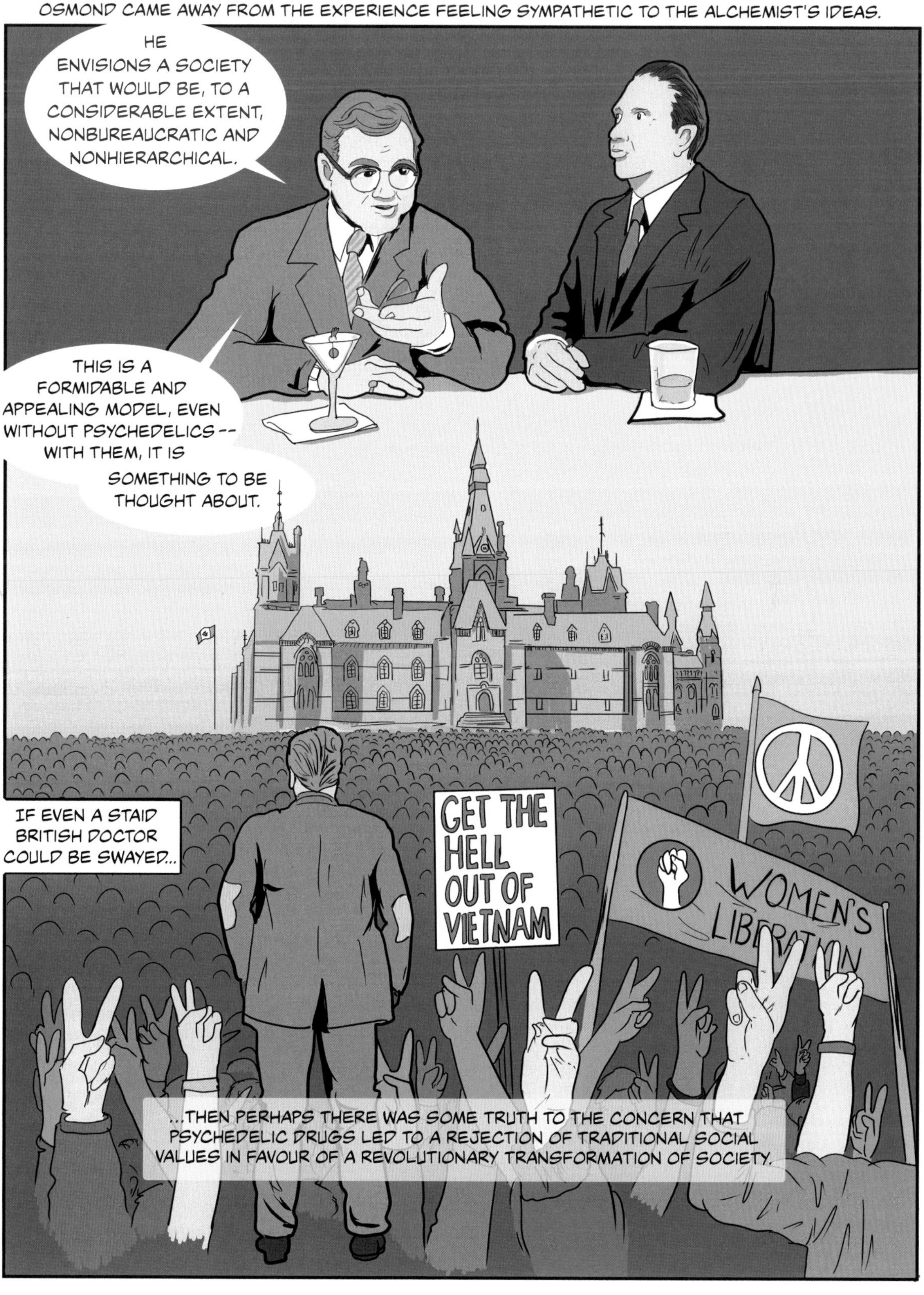
OSMOND CAME AWAY FROM THE EXPERIENCE FEELING SYMPATHETIC TO THE ALCHEMIST'S IDEAS.
HE ENVISIONS A SOCIETY THAT WOULD BE, TO A CONSIDERABLE EXTENT, NONBUREAUCRATIC AND NONHIERARCHICAL.
THIS IS A FORMIDABLE AND APPEALING MODEL, EVEN WITHOUT PSYCHEDELICS -- WITH THEM, IT IS SOMETHING TO BE THOUGHT ABOUT.
IF EVEN A STAID BRITISH DOCTOR COULD BE SWAYED...
GET THE HELL OUT OF VIETNAM
WOMEN'S LIBERATION
...THEN PERHAPS THERE WAS SOME TRUTH TO THE CONCERN THAT PSYCHEDELIC DRUGS LED TO A REJECTION OF TRADITIONAL SOCIAL VALUES IN FAVOUR OF A REVOLUTIONARY TRANSFORMATION OF SOCIETY.

THIS MAY EXPLAIN THE MORAL PANIC THAT SEIZED THE PRESS ABOUT WHAT THEY BEGAN TO CALL "ACID."

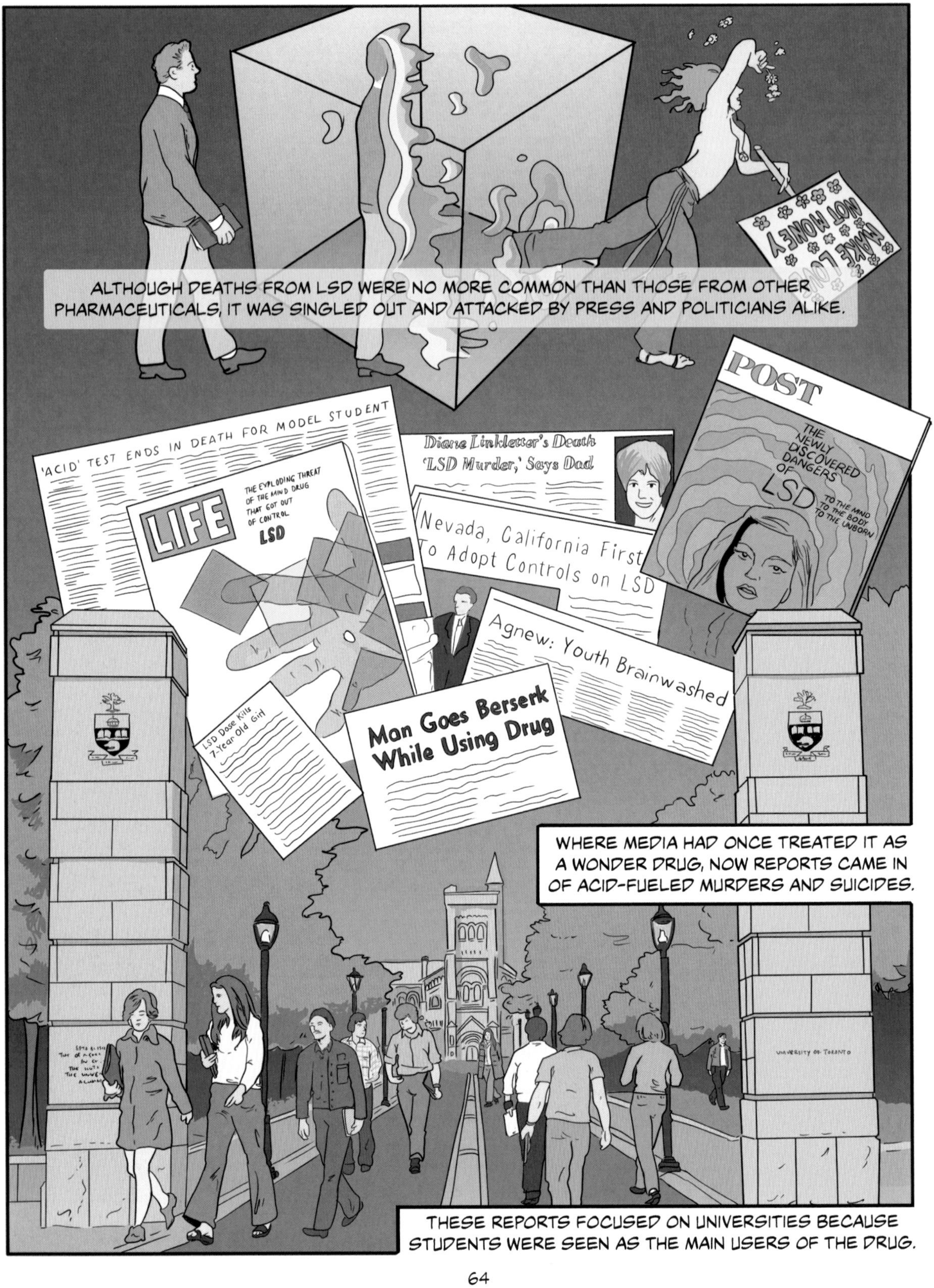
ALTHOUGH DEATHS FROM LSD WERE NO MORE COMMON THAN THOSE FROM OTHER PHARMACEUTICALS, IT WAS SINGLED OUT AND ATTACKED BY PRESS AND POLITICIANS ALIKE.
'ACID' TEST ENDS IN DEATH FOR MODEL STUDENT
LIFE
THE EXPLODING THREAT OF THE MIND DRUG THAT GOT OUT OF CONTROL
LSD
Diane Linkletter's Death 'LSD Murder,' Says Dad
POST
THE NEWLY DISCOVERED DANGERS OF LSD
TO THE MIND TO THE BODY TO THE UNBORN
Nevada, California First To Adopt Controls on LSD
Agnew: Youth Brainwashed
LSD Dose Kills 7-Year Old Girl
Man Goes Berserk While Using Drug
WHERE MEDIA HAD ONCE TREATED IT AS A WONDER DRUG, NOW REPORTS CAME IN OF ACID-FUELED MURDERS AND SUICIDES.
UNIVERSITY OF TORONTO
THESE REPORTS FOCUSED ON UNIVERSITIES BECAUSE STUDENTS WERE SEEN AS THE MAIN USERS OF THE DRUG.

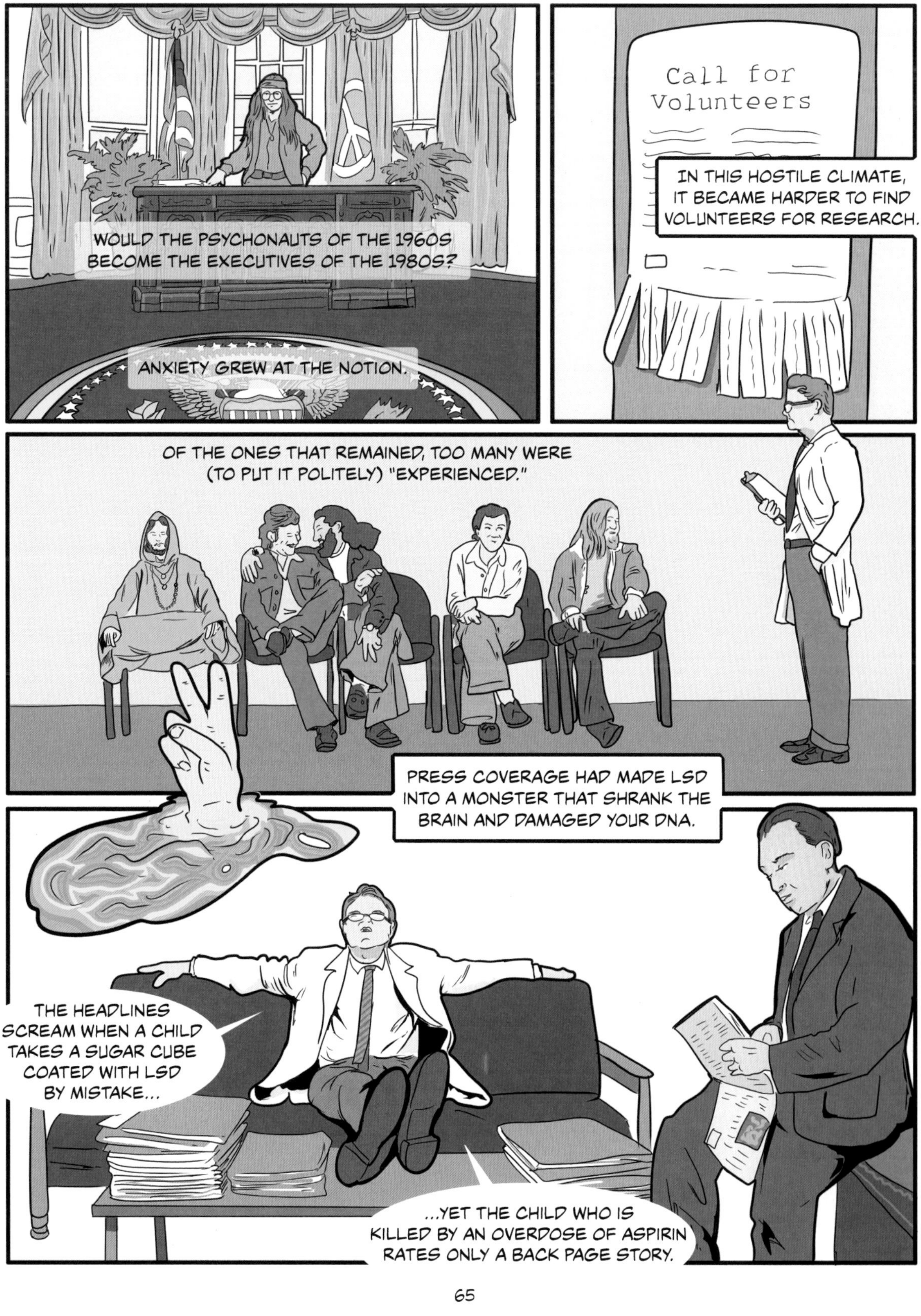
WOULD THE PSYCHONAUTS OF THE 1960S BECOME THE EXECUTIVES OF THE 1980S?
ANXIETY GREW AT THE NOTION.
Call for Volunteers
IN THIS HOSTILE CLIMATE, IT BECAME HARDER TO FIND VOLUNTEERS FOR RESEARCH.
OF THE ONES THAT REMAINED, TOO MANY WERE (TO PUT IT POLITELY) "EXPERIENCED."
PRESS COVERAGE HAD MADE LSD INTO A MONSTER THAT SHRANK THE BRAIN AND DAMAGED YOUR DNA.
THE HEADLINES SCREAM WHEN A CHILD TAKES A SUGAR CUBE COATED WITH LSD BY MISTAKE...
...YET THE CHILD WHO IS KILLED BY AN OVERDOSE OF ASPIRIN RATES ONLY A BACK PAGE STORY.

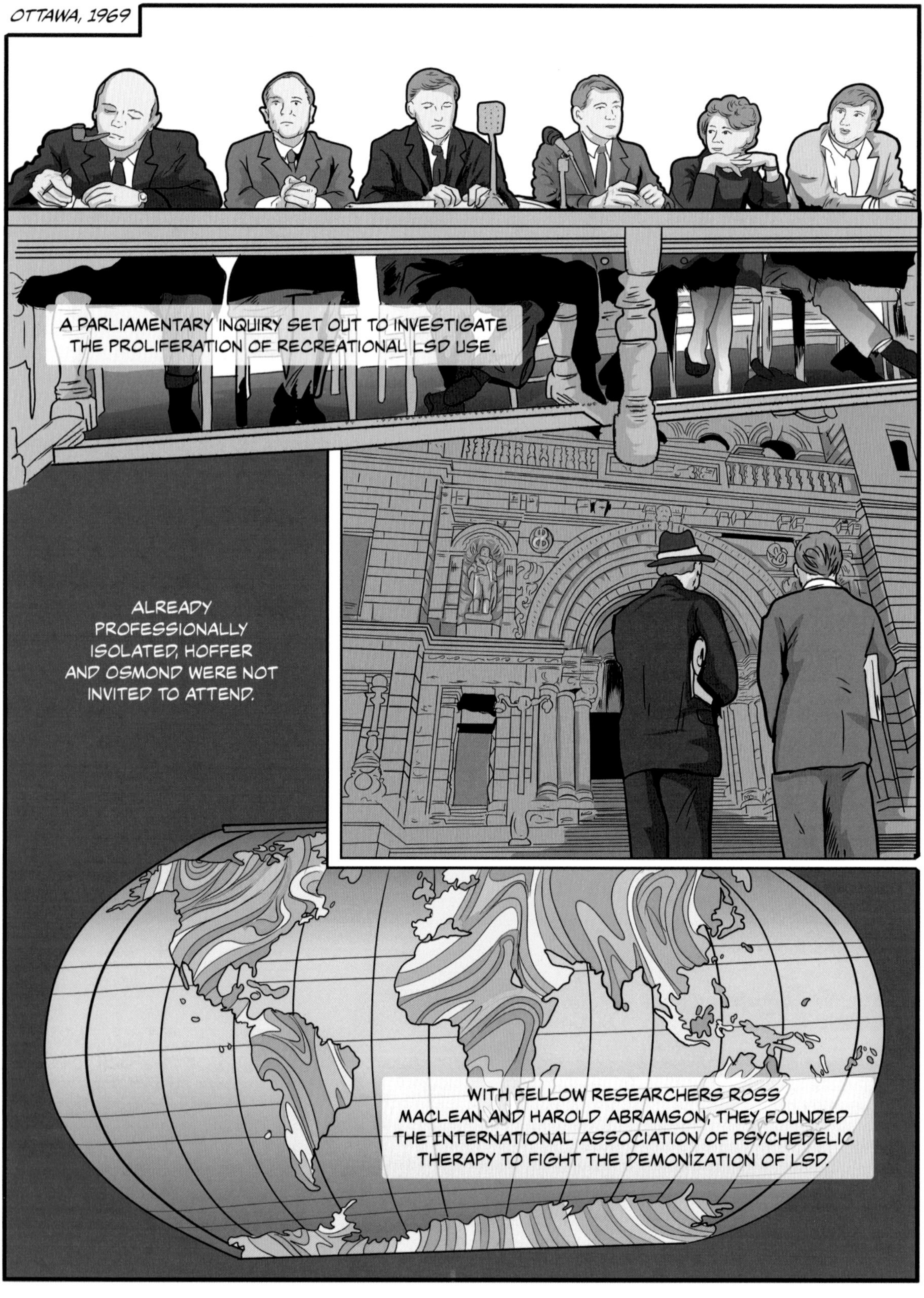
OTTAWA, 1969
A PARLIAMENTARY INQUIRY SET OUT TO INVESTIGATE THE PROLIFERATION OF RECREATIONAL LSD USE.
ALREADY PROFESSIONALLY ISOLATED, HOFFER AND OSMOND WERE NOT INVITED TO ATTEND.
WITH FELLOW RESEARCHERS ROSS MACLEAN AND HAROLD ABRAMSON, THEY FOUNDED THE INTERNATIONAL ASSOCIATION OF PSYCHEDELIC THERAPY TO FIGHT THE DEMONIZATION OF LSD.

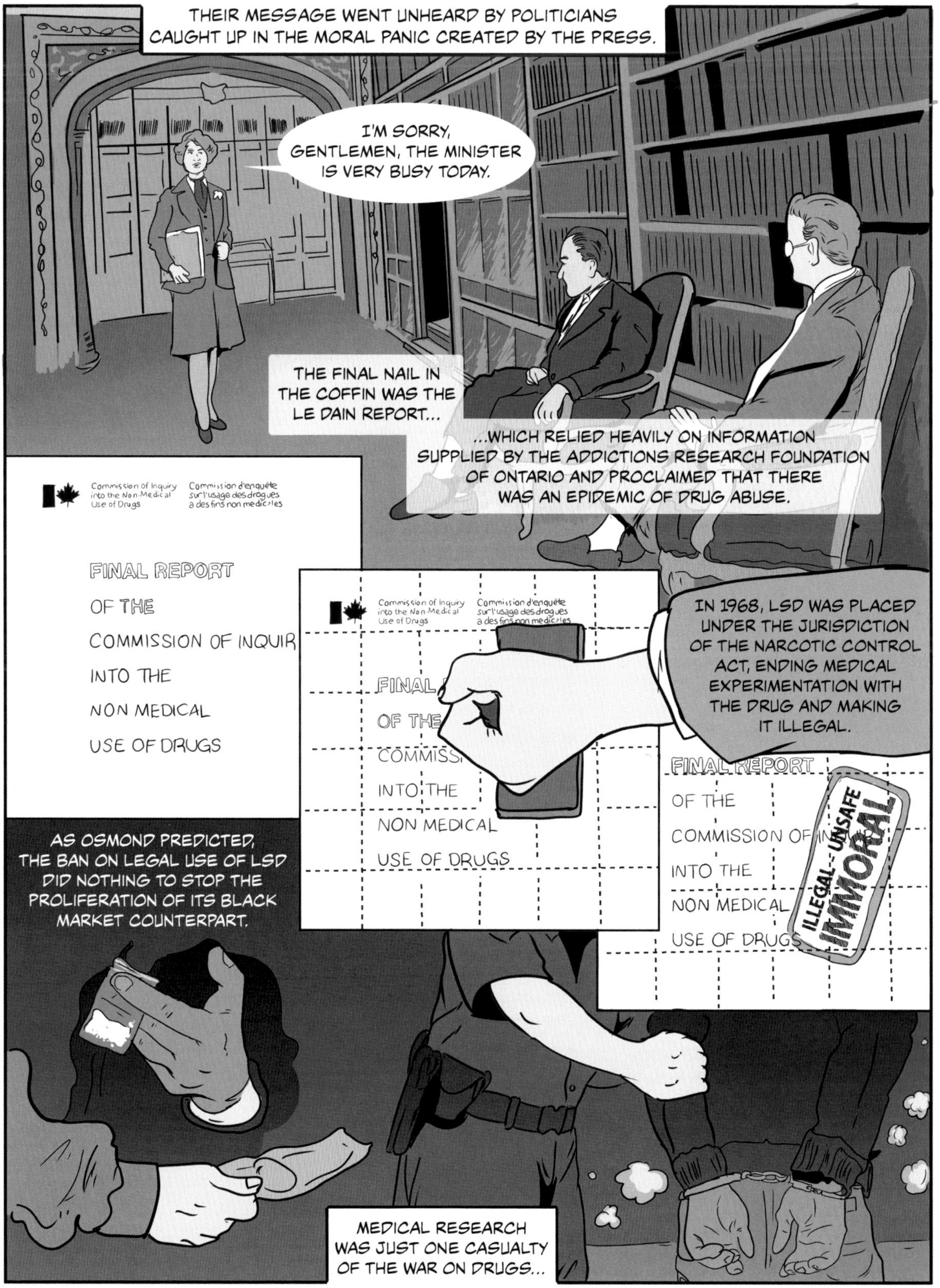
THEIR MESSAGE WENT UNHEARD BY POLITICIANS CAUGHT UP IN THE MORAL PANIC CREATED BY THE PRESS.
I'M SORRY, GENTLEMEN, THE MINISTER IS VERY BUSY TODAY.
THE FINAL NAIL IN THE COFFIN WAS THE LE DAIN REPORT...
...WHICH RELIED HEAVILY ON INFORMATION SUPPLIED BY THE ADDICTIONS RESEARCH FOUNDATION OF ONTARIO AND PROCLAIMED THAT THERE WAS AN EPIDEMIC OF DRUG ABUSE.
Commission of Inquiry into the Non-Medical Use of Drugs
Commission d'enquête sur l'usage des drogues à des fins non médicales
FINAL REPORT
OF THE
COMMISSION OF INQUIR
INTO THE
NON MEDICAL
USE OF DRUGS
IN 1968, LSD WAS PLACED UNDER THE JURISDICTION OF THE NARCOTIC CONTROL ACT, ENDING MEDICAL EXPERIMENTATION WITH THE DRUG AND MAKING IT ILLEGAL.
ILLEGAL - UNSAFE
IMMORAL
AS OSMOND PREDICTED, THE BAN ON LEGAL USE OF LSD DID NOTHING TO STOP THE PROLIFERATION OF ITS BLACK MARKET COUNTERPART.
MEDICAL RESEARCH WAS JUST ONE CASUALTY OF THE WAR ON DRUGS...

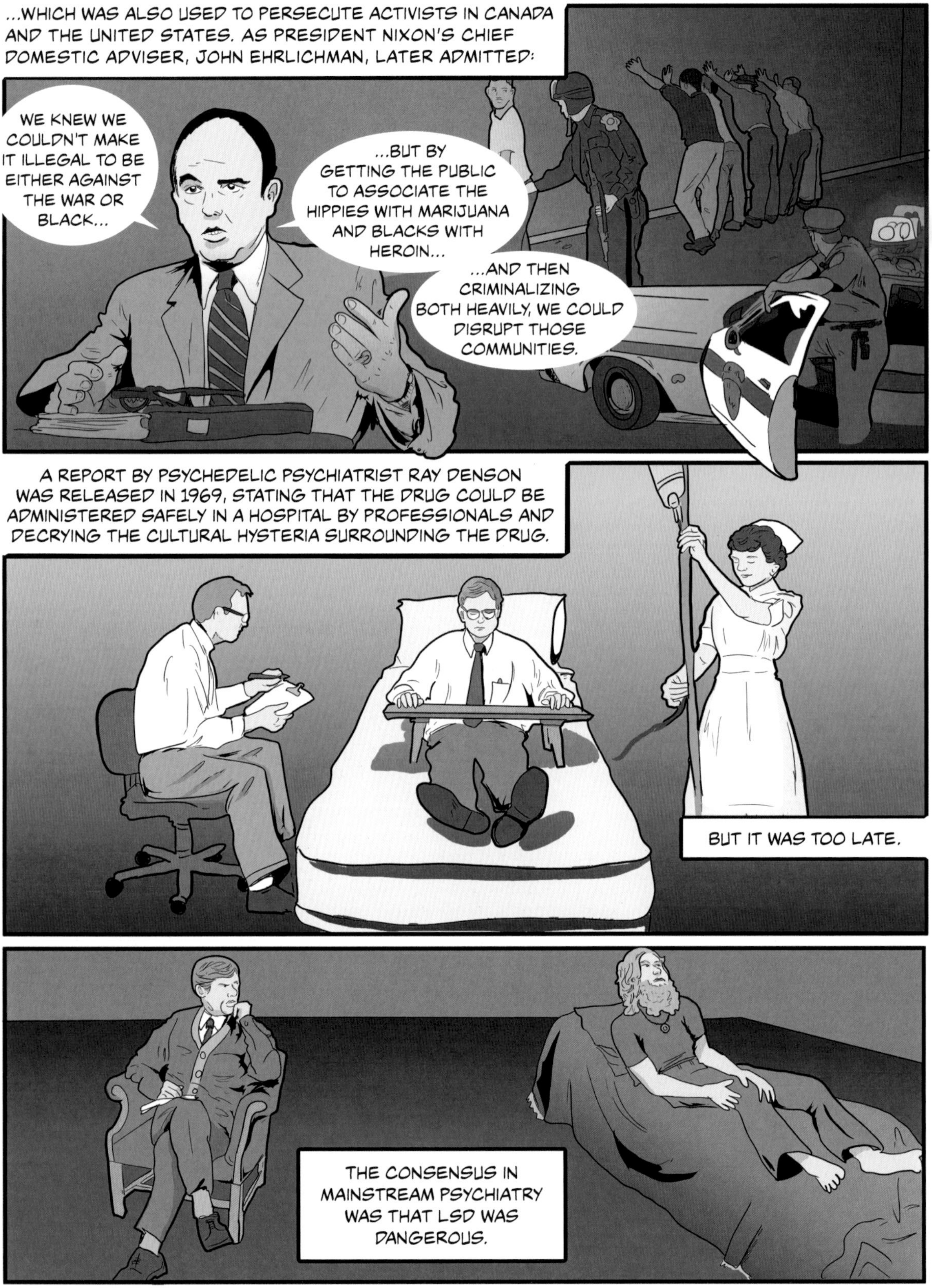
...WHICH WAS ALSO USED TO PERSECUTE ACTIVISTS IN CANADA AND THE UNITED STATES. AS PRESIDENT NIXON'S CHIEF DOMESTIC ADVISER, JOHN EHRLICHMAN, LATER ADMITTED:
WE KNEW WE COULDN'T MAKE IT ILLEGAL TO BE EITHER AGAINST THE WAR OR BLACK...
...BUT BY GETTING THE PUBLIC TO ASSOCIATE THE HIPPIES WITH MARIJUANA AND BLACKS WITH HEROIN...
...AND THEN CRIMINALIZING BOTH HEAVILY, WE COULD DISRUPT THOSE COMMUNITIES.
A REPORT BY PSYCHEDELIC PSYCHIATRIST RAY DENSON WAS RELEASED IN 1969, STATING THAT THE DRUG COULD BE ADMINISTERED SAFELY IN A HOSPITAL BY PROFESSIONALS AND DECRYING THE CULTURAL HYSTERIA SURROUNDING THE DRUG.
BUT IT WAS TOO LATE.
THE CONSENSUS IN MAINSTREAM PSYCHIATRY WAS THAT LSD WAS DANGEROUS.

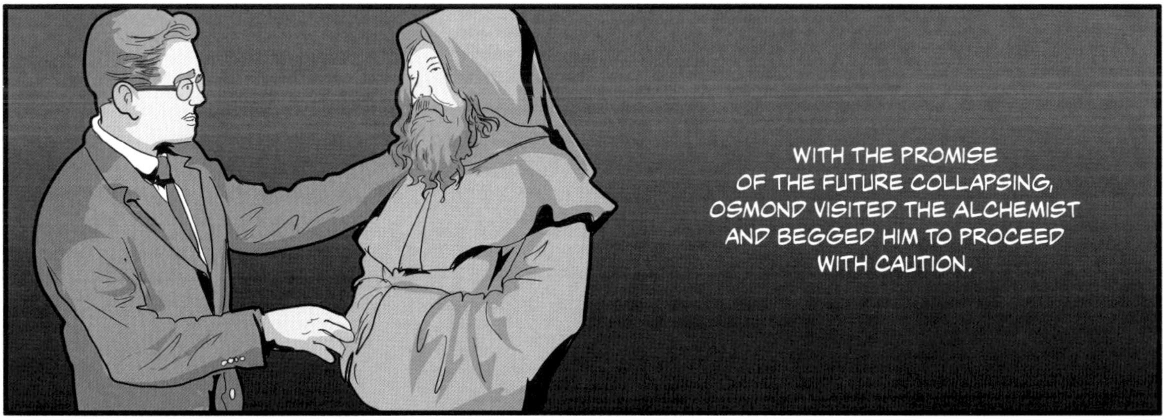
WITH THE PROMISE OF THE FUTURE COLLAPSING, OSMOND VISITED THE ALCHEMIST AND BEGGED HIM TO PROCEED WITH CAUTION.

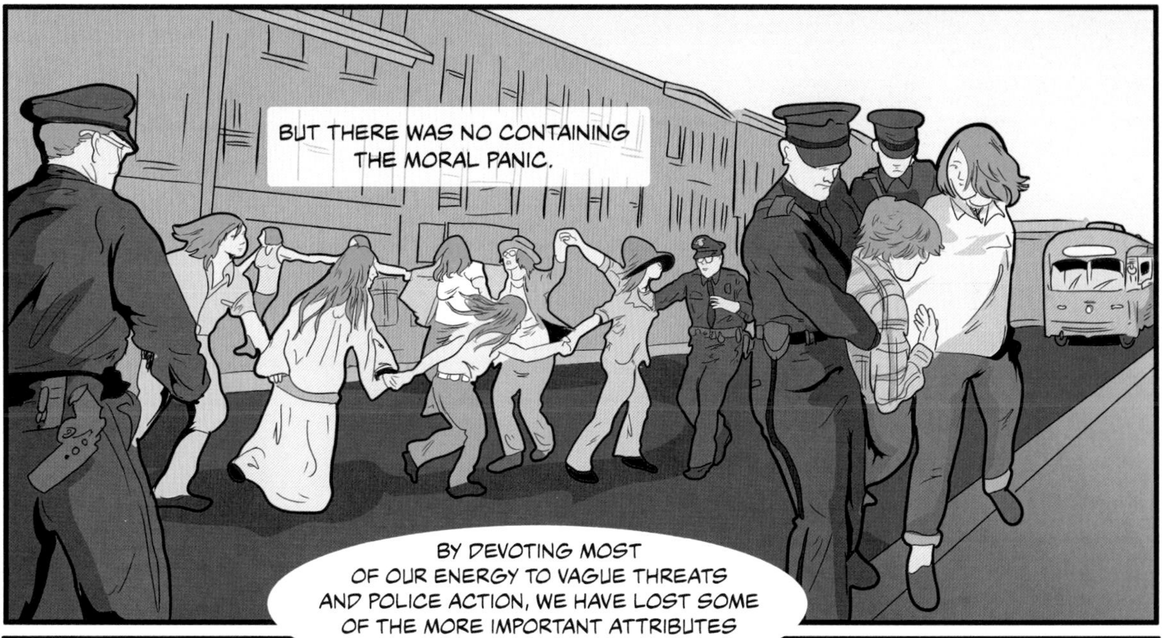
BUT THERE WAS NO CONTAINING THE MORAL PANIC.
BY DEVOTING MOST OF OUR ENERGY TO VAGUE THREATS AND POLICE ACTION, WE HAVE LOST SOME OF THE MORE IMPORTANT ATTRIBUTES OF MEDICAL AUTHORITY...

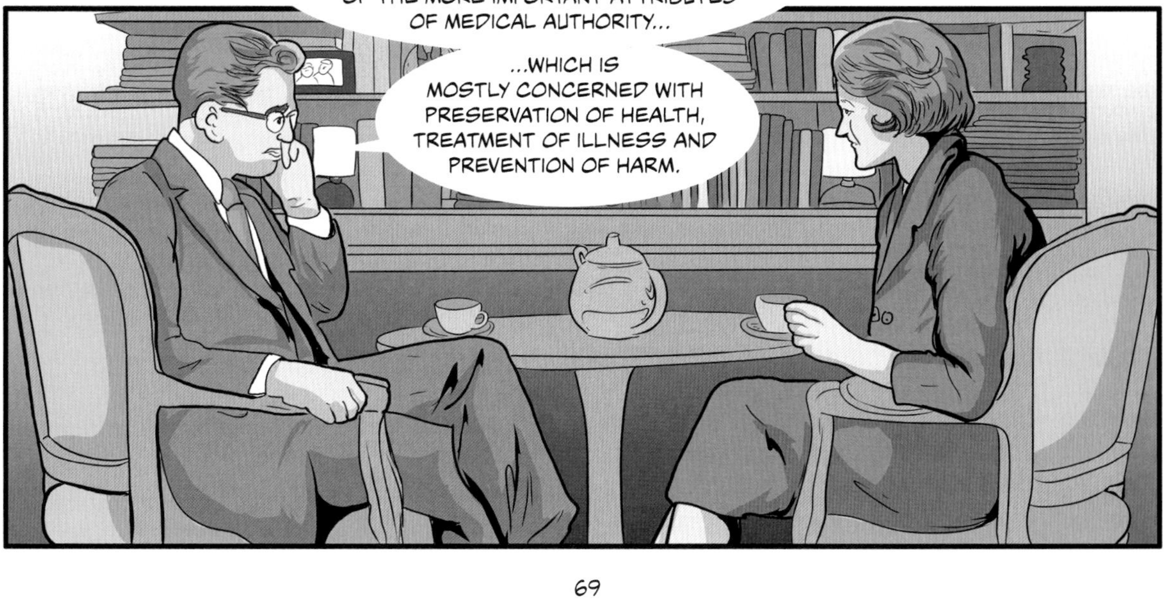
...WHICH IS MOSTLY CONCERNED WITH PRESERVATION OF HEALTH, TREATMENT OF ILLNESS AND PREVENTION OF HARM.

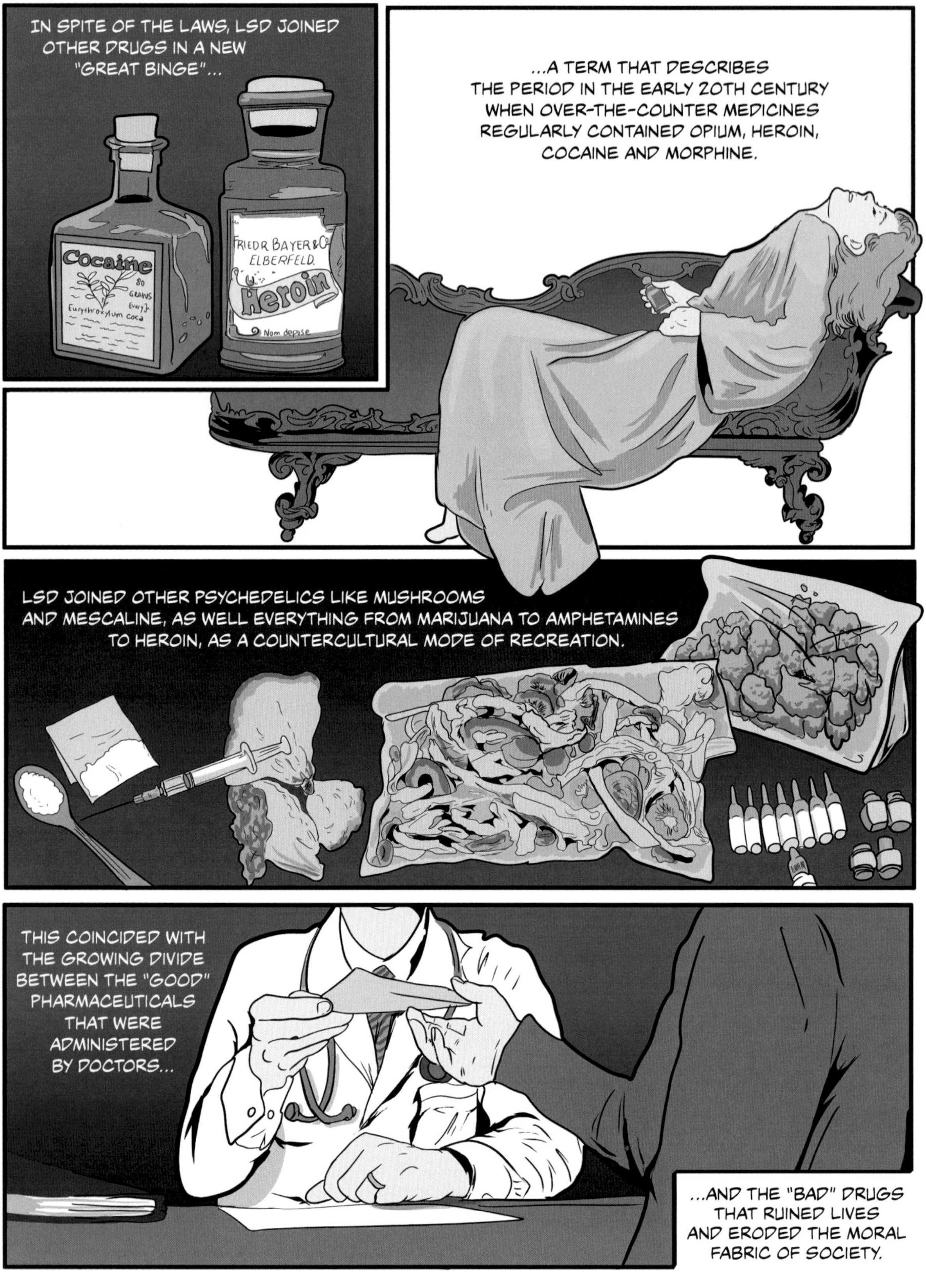
IN SPITE OF THE LAWS, LSD JOINED OTHER DRUGS IN A NEW "GREAT BINGE"...
Cocaine
80 GRAINS
Erythroxylum coca
FRIEDR BAYER & Co
ELBERFELD.
Heroin
Nom depose
...A TERM THAT DESCRIBES THE PERIOD IN THE EARLY 20TH CENTURY WHEN OVER-THE-COUNTER MEDICINES REGULARLY CONTAINED OPIUM, HEROIN, COCAINE AND MORPHINE.
LSD JOINED OTHER PSYCHEDELICS LIKE MUSHROOMS AND MESCALINE, AS WELL EVERYTHING FROM MARIJUANA TO AMPHETAMINES TO HEROIN, AS A COUNTERCULTURAL MODE OF RECREATION.
THIS COINCIDED WITH THE GROWING DIVIDE BETWEEN THE "GOOD" PHARMACEUTICALS THAT WERE ADMINISTERED BY DOCTORS...
...AND THE "BAD" DRUGS THAT RUINED LIVES AND ERODED THE MORAL FABRIC OF SOCIETY.

AFTER LESS THAN 20 YEARS AS A SERIOUS RESEARCH SUBJECT...

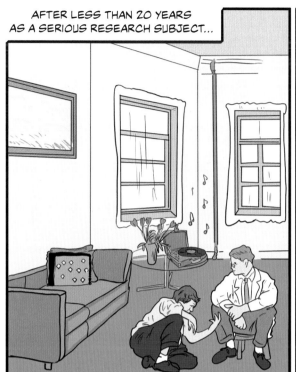

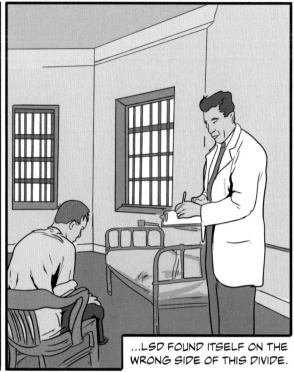

...LSD FOUND ITSELF ON THE WRONG SIDE OF THIS DIVIDE.

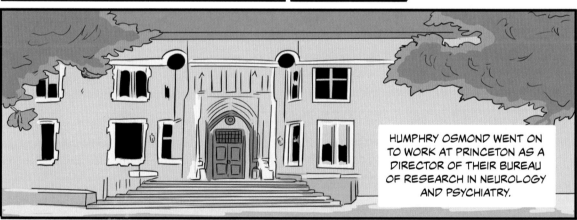

HUMPHRY OSMOND WENT ON TO WORK AT PRINCETON AS A DIRECTOR OF THEIR BUREAU OF RESEARCH IN NEUROLOGY AND PSYCHIATRY.

IN SPITE OF HIS FEARS THAT HE MIGHT BE REMEMBERED AS "THE MAN WHO DROVE ALDOUS HUXLEY MAD," HIS MOST LASTING LEGACY WAS COINING THE TERM "PSYCHEDELIC"...

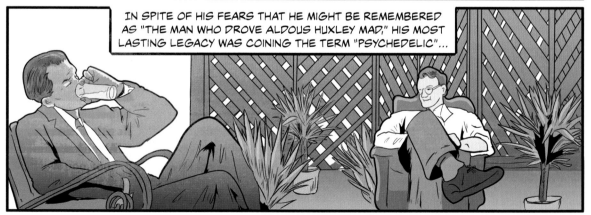

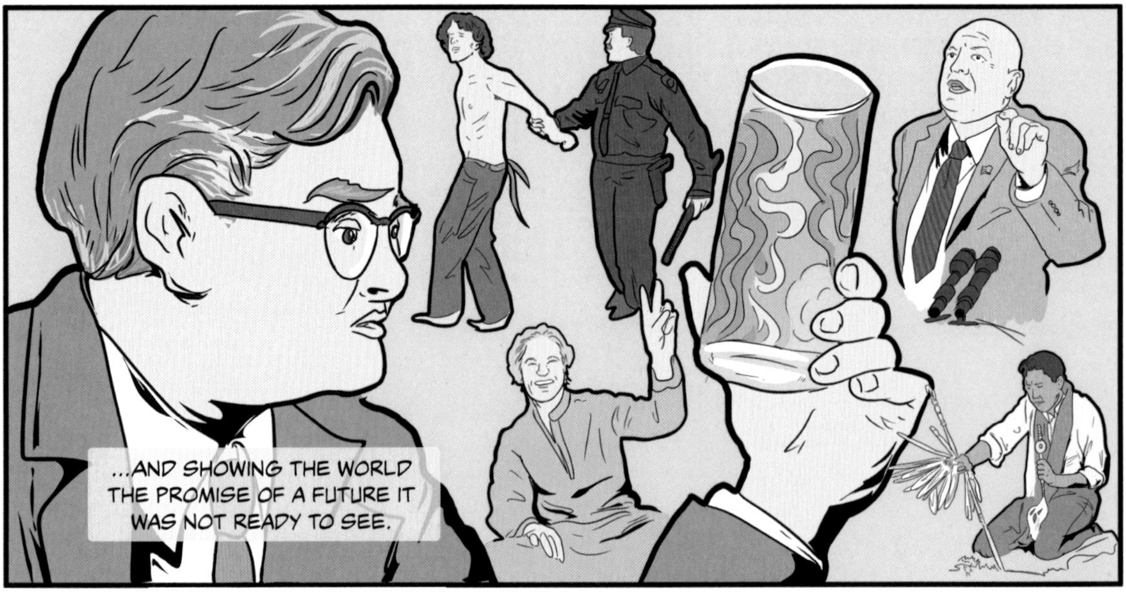
...AND SHOWING THE WORLD THE PROMISE OF A FUTURE IT WAS NOT READY TO SEE.

IN 1970, ONE OF CHARLES MANSON'S FOLLOWERS ATTEMPTED TO POISON A WITNESS IN HIS TRIAL BY PUTTING 10 HITS OF ACID IN A HAMBURGER.*

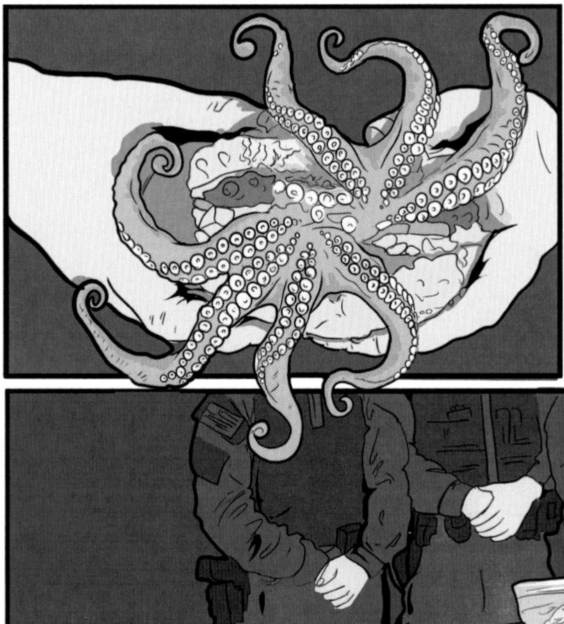

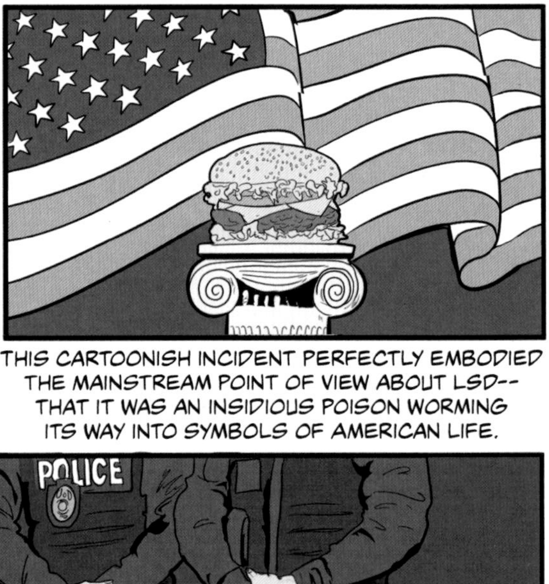

THIS CARTOONISH INCIDENT PERFECTLY EMBODIED THE MAINSTREAM POINT OF VIEW ABOUT LSD--THAT IT WAS AN INSIDIOUS POISON WORMING ITS WAY INTO SYMBOLS OF AMERICAN LIFE.

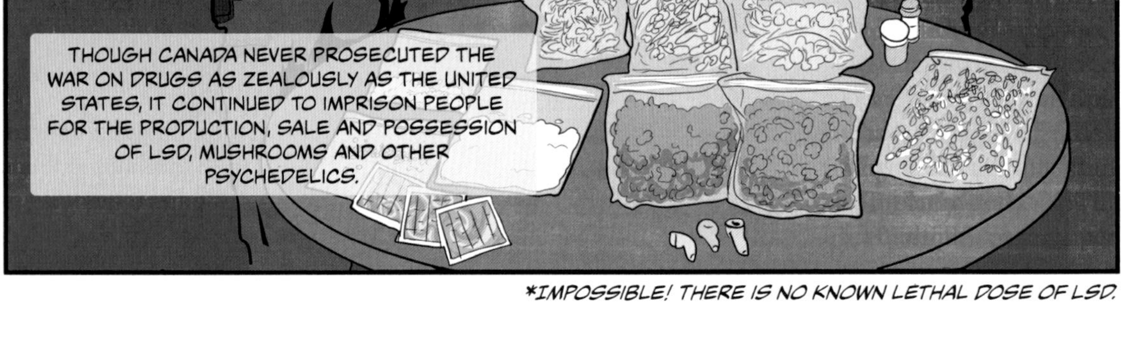
POLICE
THOUGH CANADA NEVER PROSECUTED THE WAR ON DRUGS AS ZEALOUSLY AS THE UNITED STATES, IT CONTINUED TO IMPRISON PEOPLE FOR THE PRODUCTION, SALE AND POSSESSION OF LSD, MUSHROOMS AND OTHER PSYCHEDELICS.

*IMPOSSIBLE! THERE IS NO KNOWN LETHAL DOSE OF LSD.

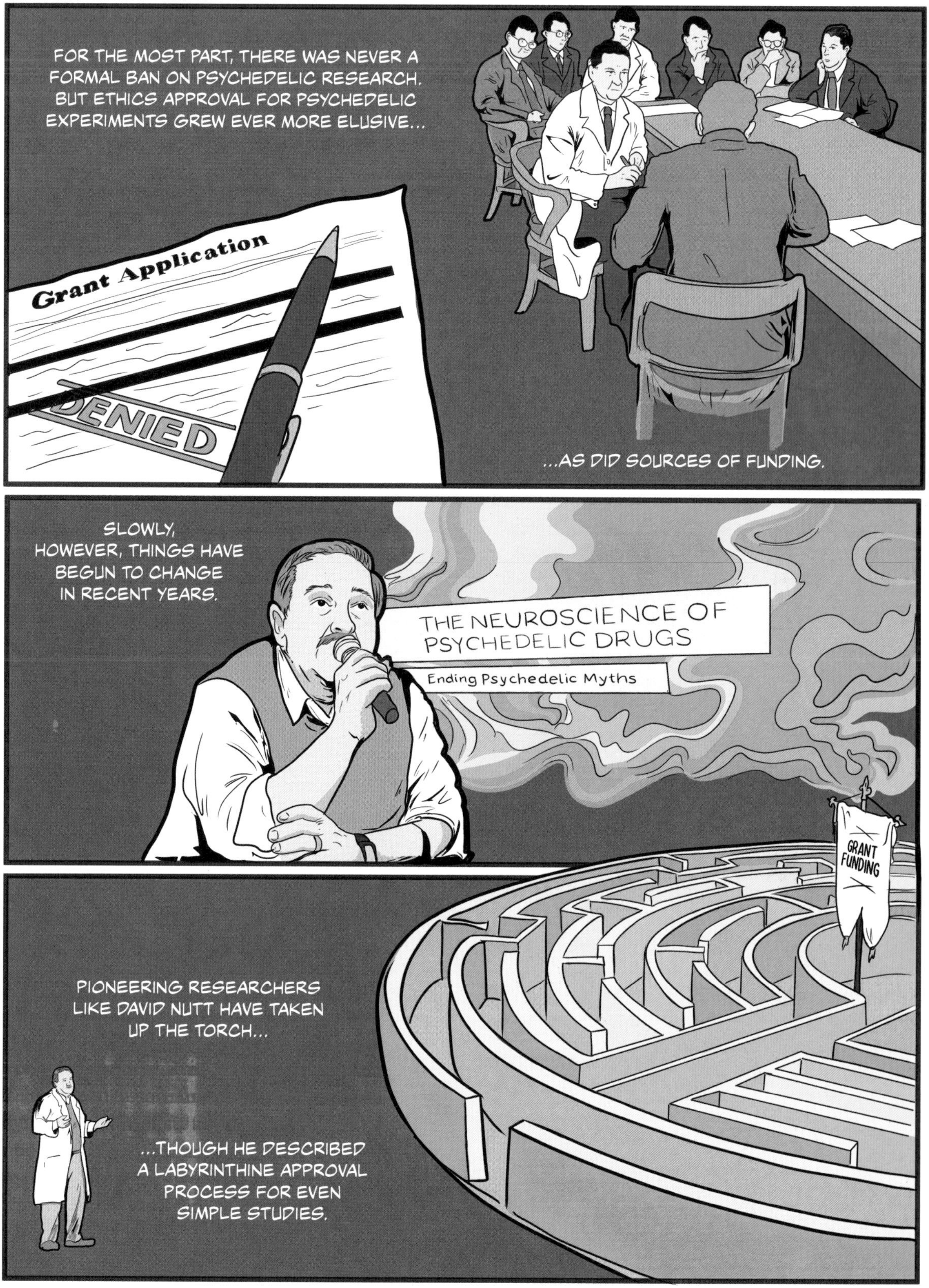
FOR THE MOST PART, THERE WAS NEVER A FORMAL BAN ON PSYCHEDELIC RESEARCH. BUT ETHICS APPROVAL FOR PSYCHEDELIC EXPERIMENTS GREW EVER MORE ELUSIVE...
Grant Application
DENIED
...AS DID SOURCES OF FUNDING.
SLOWLY, HOWEVER, THINGS HAVE BEGUN TO CHANGE IN RECENT YEARS.
THE NEUROSCIENCE OF PSYCHEDELIC DRUGS
Ending Psychedelic Myths
GRANT FUNDING
PIONEERING RESEARCHERS LIKE DAVID NUTT HAVE TAKEN UP THE TORCH...
...THOUGH HE DESCRIBED A LABYRINTHINE APPROVAL PROCESS FOR EVEN SIMPLE STUDIES.

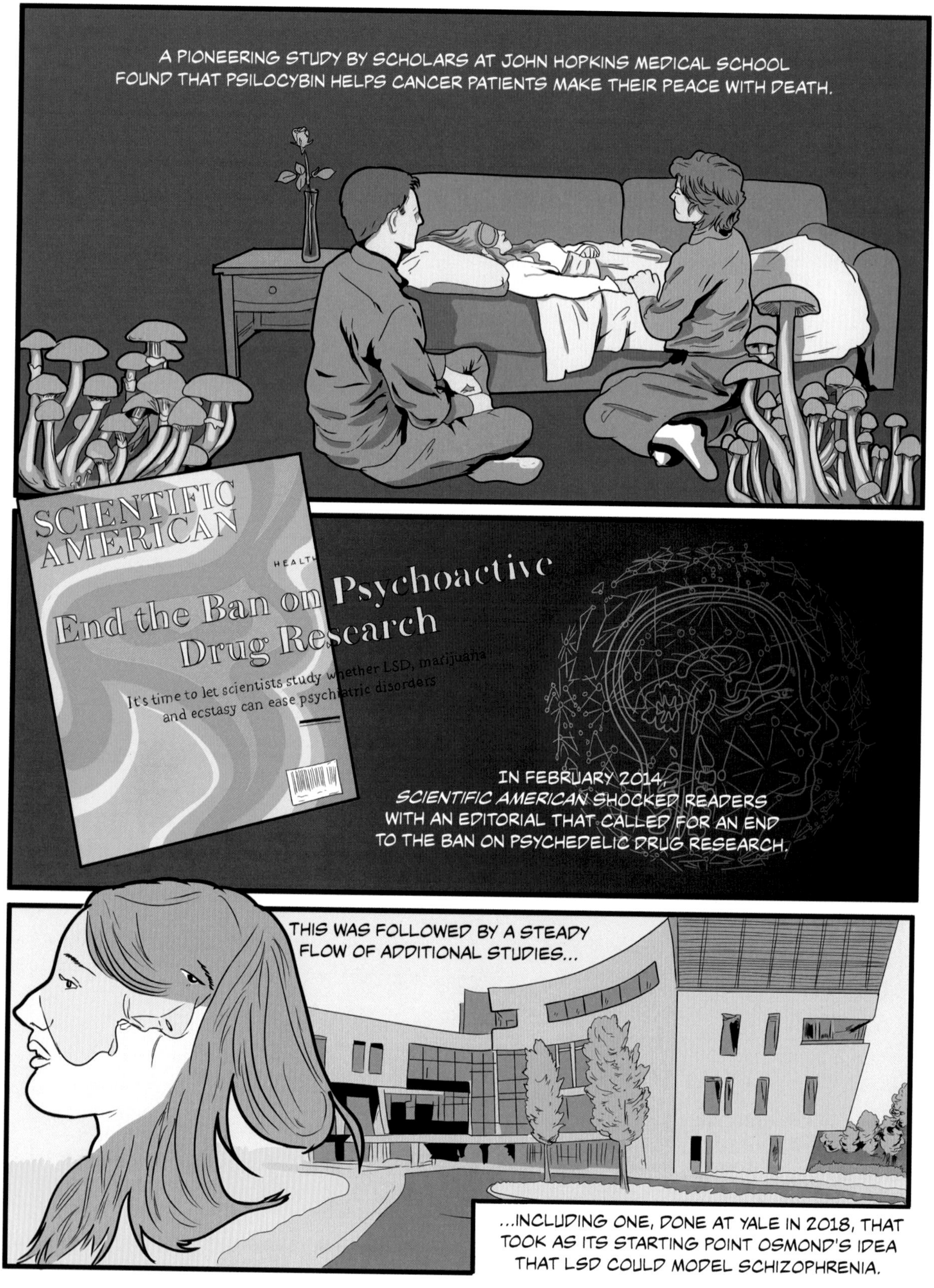
A PIONEERING STUDY BY SCHOLARS AT JOHN HOPKINS MEDICAL SCHOOL FOUND THAT PSILOCYBIN HELPS CANCER PATIENTS MAKE THEIR PEACE WITH DEATH.
SCIENTIFIC AMERICAN
HEALTH
End the Ban on Psychoactive Drug Research
It's time to let scientists study whether LSD, marijuana and ecstasy can ease psychiatric disorders
IN FEBRUARY 2014, *SCIENTIFIC AMERICAN* SHOCKED READERS WITH AN EDITORIAL THAT CALLED FOR AN END TO THE BAN ON PSYCHEDELIC DRUG RESEARCH.
THIS WAS FOLLOWED BY A STEADY FLOW OF ADDITIONAL STUDIES...
...INCLUDING ONE, DONE AT YALE IN 2018, THAT TOOK AS ITS STARTING POINT OSMOND'S IDEA THAT LSD COULD MODEL SCHIZOPHRENIA.

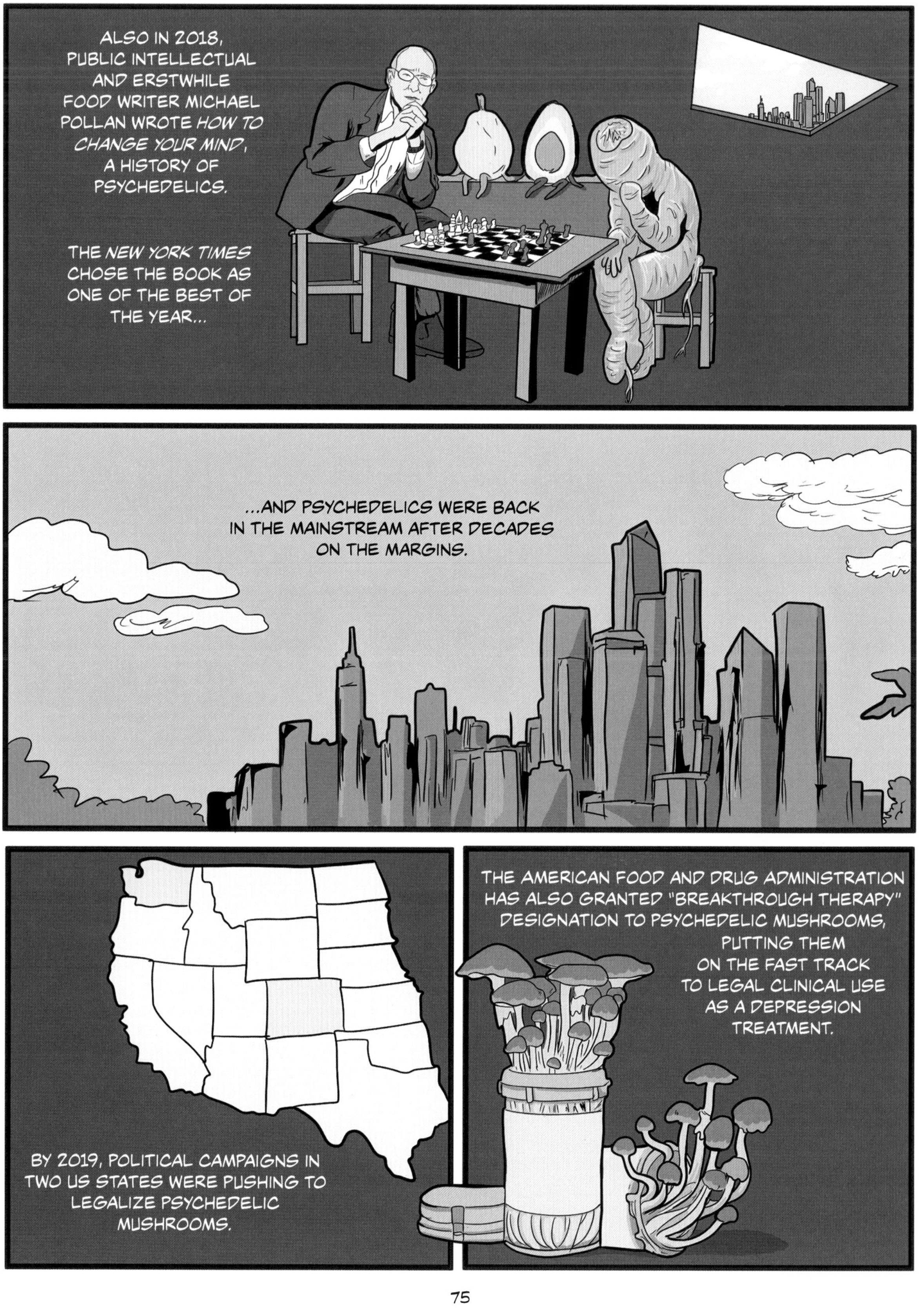
ALSO IN 2018, PUBLIC INTELLECTUAL AND ERSTWHILE FOOD WRITER MICHAEL POLLAN WROTE *HOW TO CHANGE YOUR MIND*, A HISTORY OF PSYCHEDELICS.
THE *NEW YORK TIMES* CHOSE THE BOOK AS ONE OF THE BEST OF THE YEAR...
...AND PSYCHEDELICS WERE BACK IN THE MAINSTREAM AFTER DECADES ON THE MARGINS.
BY 2019, POLITICAL CAMPAIGNS IN TWO US STATES WERE PUSHING TO LEGALIZE PSYCHEDELIC MUSHROOMS.
THE AMERICAN FOOD AND DRUG ADMINISTRATION HAS ALSO GRANTED "BREAKTHROUGH THERAPY" DESIGNATION TO PSYCHEDELIC MUSHROOMS, PUTTING THEM ON THE FAST TRACK TO LEGAL CLINICAL USE AS A DEPRESSION TREATMENT.

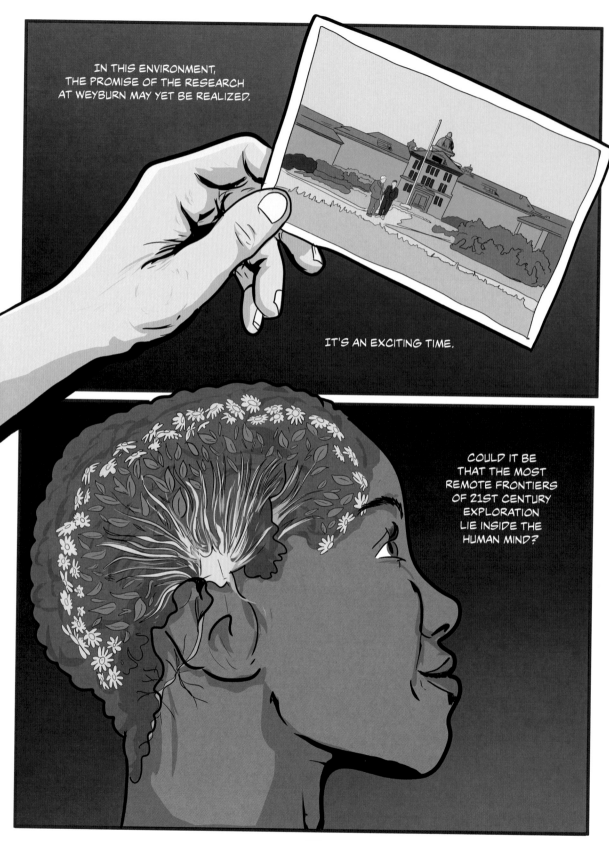

IN THIS ENVIRONMENT, THE PROMISE OF THE RESEARCH AT WEYBURN MAY YET BE REALIZED.

IT'S AN EXCITING TIME.

COULD IT BE THAT THE MOST REMOTE FRONTIERS OF 21ST CENTURY EXPLORATION LIE INSIDE THE HUMAN MIND?

Psychedelic Pasts

A Trip to be Remembered

Dr. Erika Dyck

In 1994 I met Timothy Leary. I was still a teenager, freshly enrolled at the University of Saskatchewan and working at a student-run movie theatre where Leary was scheduled to speak. My job was to show him around, get him water, make sure his microphone worked. He asked for popcorn with extra butter before he went on stage. I was struck by the sizeable liver spots dotting his arms, his slightly shaking hands, but above all his twinkling eyes and ever-present smile. Talking to him was effortless, whether about popcorn or the weather. He looked right at me and spoke to me as though my opinions on butter mattered, even though I was a shy student employee mostly trying to be invisible. I had no idea who this guy was or why the event was sold out. But I led him to the stage certain that I had just learned what it meant to have charisma—this guy oozed it.

In the days before the world-wide-web I suppose I could have gone to the library to find out more about who this Timothy Leary guy was in preparation for his visit. Saskatoon, Saskatchewan, is not typically known as a hot spot for touring speakers, and I think I assumed he was just another academic passing through. Had I visited the library in that pre-Internet era I would have had to dig to find out very much about Leary. He had published some scientific papers and co-founded the *Psychedelic Review*, but without knowing his connection to psychedelics it is unlikely I would have stumbled upon these details in the card catalogue. I would have had to visit the newspaper microfilm reading room and scroll through unindexed films to discover his countercultural fame and popularity—but then again, only if I had known where to look. But I didn't do any of this.

Leary took the stage and dazzled the audience, in an otherwise dark theatre, with a lightshow and accompanying soundscape. His voice carried messages of love, inspiration, and mind freedom. To be honest, I was confused. I had no idea what he was talking about or why the crowd was bathed in a kaleidoscopic light show. I was surprised when he thanked the good people of Saskatchewan at the end of his presentation, and I watched other puzzled audience members file out of the auditorium after the rather bizarre presentation.

Two years later I read that Timothy Leary had died and that he had requested that his ashes be catapulted into space so he could continue his epic journey.

I didn't realize it at the time, but in some ways meeting Leary in Saskatchewan sent me on my own epic journey. Mine would be much less colourful—decidedly monochromatic, in fact—and filled with boxes of photocopies, microfilm reels of news stories, and handwritten notes about medical experiments. Much like most of my classmates at the University of Saskatchewan in the 1990s, I had no idea that the province had been home to a wide range of LSD and mescaline experiments in the 1950s, resulting, perhaps most famously, in the coining of the term *psychedelic*.

Scientists, botanists, anthropologists, psychiatrists, and philosophers—to name a few—have had a long-standing interest in mind alteration and the kinds of substances that alter the filters in our consciousness. Aldous Huxley, after trying mescaline, described these drugs as capable of opening "doors of perception" or changing the way we think about or know ourselves. Since at least the 1920s scientists and botanists working with psychoactive plant compounds have been keen to separate these drugs from their cultural, spiritual, and healing contexts. In laboratory and clinical settings, researchers—including, notably, Timothy Leary—began establishing guidelines for creating the right environment for optimizing the effects of psychedelics, a concept Leary called "set and setting." By this he and others meant that those taking psychedelics needed to respect the experience by preparing themselves for it. This involved carefully preparing the physical environment in which the experience would take place and choreographing its emotional temperament by determining who should be present. Details from the artwork and music to the carpet were carefully selected as psychedelic adventurers reflected on their lives in anticipation of an experience that might cause them to see themselves differently.

While western-trained researchers established rules for psychedelic therapies aimed at changing behaviours—from alcoholism to sexual disorders—anthropologists readily recognized that Indigenous ways of knowing these plant-based medicines combined ceremony, spirituality, and healing. Some clinical investigators, like Humphry Osmond, who is featured in this book, eagerly observed these practices and reflected on the importance of ritual, meditation, and deference in the use of psychedelics. These medicines, he felt, demanded respect and were not designed for casual use—or in his words, "kicks."

Leary came to embody—even champion—a different way of using psychedelics. He was not alone, but he became a key proponent of a psychedelic ethos that merged with a growing social movement whose mantra was power to the people. Psychedelics in the hands of everyone promised a very different future than psychedelics only in the hands of a credentialed few. The countercultural embrace of psychedelics changed the storyline dramatically. The proverbial genie was out of the bottle, and psychedelic drugs became a controversial medicine. A drug treatment that required coordination with music, flowers, and artwork and sometimes hallucinations to bring about therapeutic benefits was hardly a typical or cost-efficient approach to managing mental illness, especially when compared to newly introduced anti-depressants, which offered a discrete tablet for personal, daily use. Meanwhile, psychedelic use for individual mind freedom, creative expression, and personal exploration fed western appetites for social reforms aimed at elevating individual choices over social reforms that challenged systems of oppression, like patriarchy, heteronormativity, capitalism, or colonialism. The very idea of psychedelics became a badge of freedom from the drudgery of a conservative or status quo existence, and that message became embroidered in a Sixties aesthetic.

When I entered university in the 1990s, I was a typical Saskatchewan student. I wore a bunny-hug* and baggy clothes; I drank beer; I went to grunge concerts and occasionally smoked pot. Most of my friends stayed away from psychedelics, convinced that acid would fry your brains. None of them knew that an entirely different view of psychedelics had put Saskatchewan on the map.

Collaborating with Hugh and Nicole on this project has been immensely rewarding. We immediately shared an enthusiasm for historical accuracy combined with creative expression, and it has been truly inspiring to work

* *Bunny-hug*, a term unique to Saskatchewan, refers to what people elsewhere call a hoodie or hooded sweatshirt.

with this talented team on bringing this story to new audiences. In addition to learning about much more than Timothy Leary's preference for butter on his popcorn, my journey into the history of psychedelics has taught me that these stories matter. In the wake of decriminalization movements in the twenty-first century, we are beginning to adopt a new attitude toward drugs, rejecting "just say no" in favour of a new slogan—"just say know."

A new set of questions are emerging in the twenty-first century as regulators, health authorities, and social activists question why some drugs are considered harmful while others are promoted as medicines and why some can move across these categories. Possession of cannabis once led to jail time, for example, but it now can be purchased at a corner store and consumed both recreationally and medicinally.

On August 12, 2020, this historical journey came full circle. Saskatoon resident Thomas Hartle, a fifty-two-year-old IT specialist and father of two, took psilocybin mushrooms under medical supervision. Hartle was the first person in Canada in this century to receive permission from Health Canada to consume psychedelics for end-of-life anxiety. Hartle, like me, grew up in Saskatchewan and did not know that his cancer diagnosis would eventually lead to him playing a historic role in the continuation of a psychedelic story that is much more about exploring health benefits than it is about drug abuse and fried brains. Perhaps it is fitting that our province is shaped like a rectangle since working with psychedelics compels us to think outside the box.

Further Readings

Barber, Patrick. *Psychedelic Revolutionaries: Three Medical Pioneers, the Fall of Hallucinogenic Research and the Rise of Big Pharma*. London: Zed Books, 2019.

Bisbee, Cynthia, Paul Bisbee, Erika Dyck, Patrick Farrell, James Sexton, and Jim Spisak, eds. *Psychedelic Prophets: The Letters of Aldous Huxley and Humphry Osmond*. Montreal: McGill-Queen's University Press, 2018.

Chacruna Institute for Psychedelic Plant Medicines, https://chacruna.net/.

Dawson, Alexander. *The Peyote Effect: From the Inquisition to the War on Drugs*. Oakland: University of California Press, 2018.

Dyck, Erika. "'Hitting Highs at Rock Bottom': LSD Treatment for Alcoholism, 1950–1970." *Social History of Medicine* 19, no. 2 (August 2006): 313–329.

Dyck, Erika. *Psychedelic Psychiatry: LSD from Clinic to Campus*. Baltimore: Johns Hopkins University Press, 2008.

Dyck, Erika, and Fannie Kahan, eds. *Culture's Catalyst: Encounters with Peyote and the Native American Church in Canada*. Winnipeg: University of Manitoba Press, 2016.

Greenfield, R. *Timothy Leary: A Biography*. Orlando, FL: Harcourt, 2006.

Hagenback, Dieter, and Lucius Werthmuller. *Mystic Chemist: The Life of Albert Hofmann and His Discovery of LSD*. Santa Fe, NM: Synergetic Press, 2011.

Hartogsohn, Ido. *American Trip: Set and Setting and the Psychedelic Experience in the 20th Century.* Cambridge: The MIT Press, 2020.

Hoffer, Abram, and Humphry Osmond. *The Hallucinogens.* New York: Academic Press, Inc., 1967.

Hofmann, Albert. *LSD: My Problem Child.* New York: Oxford University Press, 2013. First published in 1979.

Jay, Mike. *Mescaline: A Global History of the First Psychedelic.* New Haven: Yale University Press, 2019.

Kinzer, Stephen. *Poisoner in Chief: Sidney Gottlieb and the CIA Search for Mind Control.* New York: Henry Holt, 2019.

Lattin, Don. *How Timothy Leary, Ram Dass, Huston Smith, and Andrew Weil Killed the Fifties and Ushered in a New Age for America.* New York: HarperOne, 2010.

Langlitz, Nicolas. *Neuropsychedelia: The Revival of Hallucinogen Research Since the Decade of the Brain.* Oakland: California Press, 2012.

Leary, Timothy, Ralph Metzner, and Richard Alpert. *The Psychedelic Experience: A Manual Based on the Tibetan Book of the Dead.* New York: Penguin Press, 2009. First published in 1964.

Lee, Martin A., and Bruce Shlain. *Acid Dreams: The Complete Social History of LSD: The CIA, the Sixties, and Beyond.* New York: Grove Press, 1985.

Oram, Matthew. *The Trials of Psychedelic Therapy: LSD Psychotherapy in America.* Baltimore: Johns Hopkins University Press, 2018.

Pollan, Michael. *How to Change Your Mind: What the New Science of Psychedelics Teaches Us About Consciousness, Dying, Addiction, Depression, and Transcendence.* New York: Penguin Press, 2017.

Richards, William. *Sacred Knowledge: Psychedelics and Religious Experiences*. New York: Columbia University Press, 2016.

Rothenberg, Jerome, ed. *Maria Sabina: Selections*. Berkley: University of California Press, 2003.

Schultz, Richard, and Albert Hofmann. *Plants of the Gods: Their Sacred, Healing and Hallucinogenic Powers*. Rochester, VT: Healing Arts, 1979.

Siff, Stephen. *Acid Hype: American News Media and the Psychedelic Experience*. Champaign: University of Illinois Press, 2015.

Stevens, Jay. *Storming Heaven: LSD and the American Dream*. New York: Grove Press, 1987.

Wasson, R. Gordon. "Seeking the Magic Mushroom." *Life*, May 13, 1957.

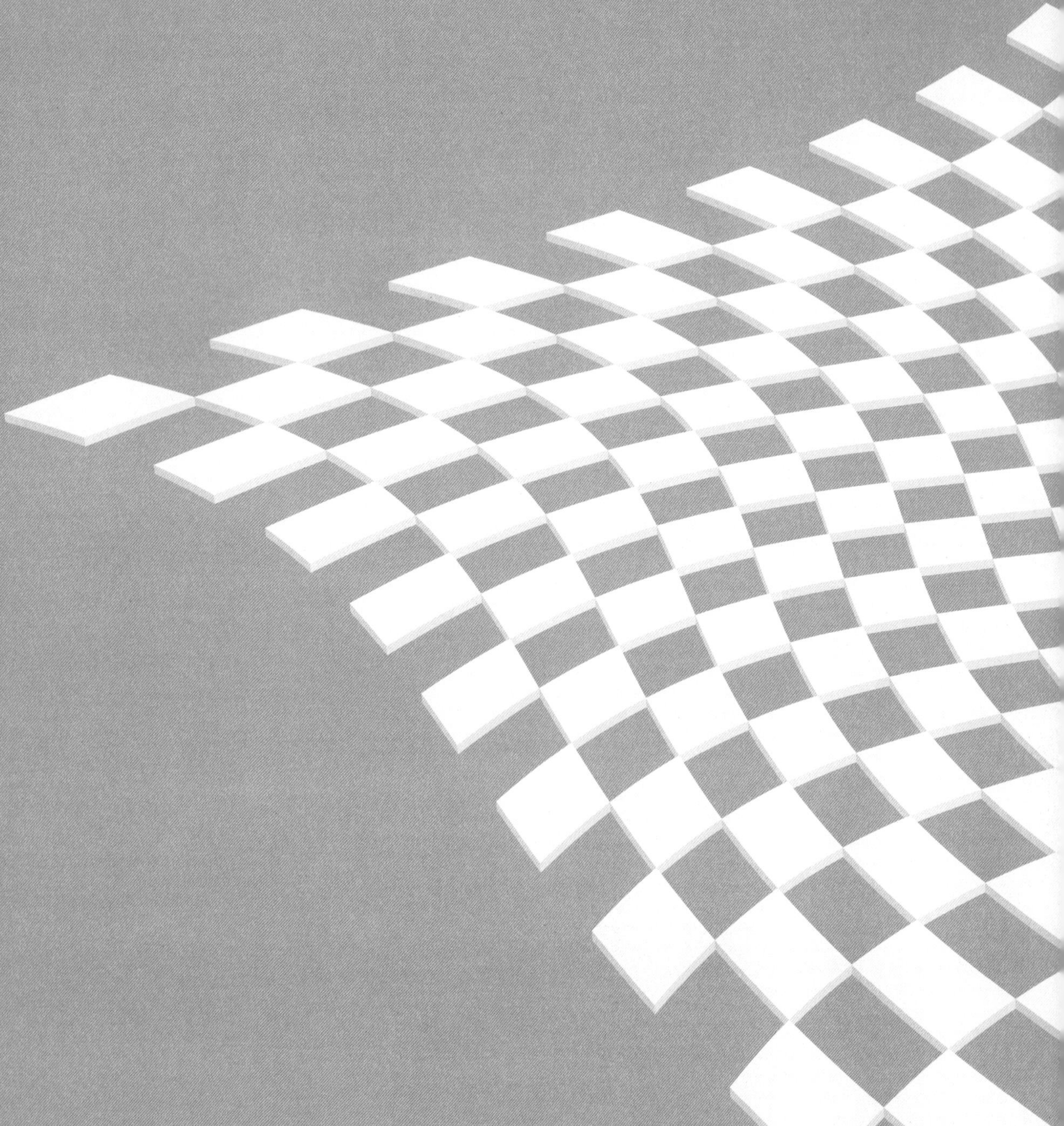

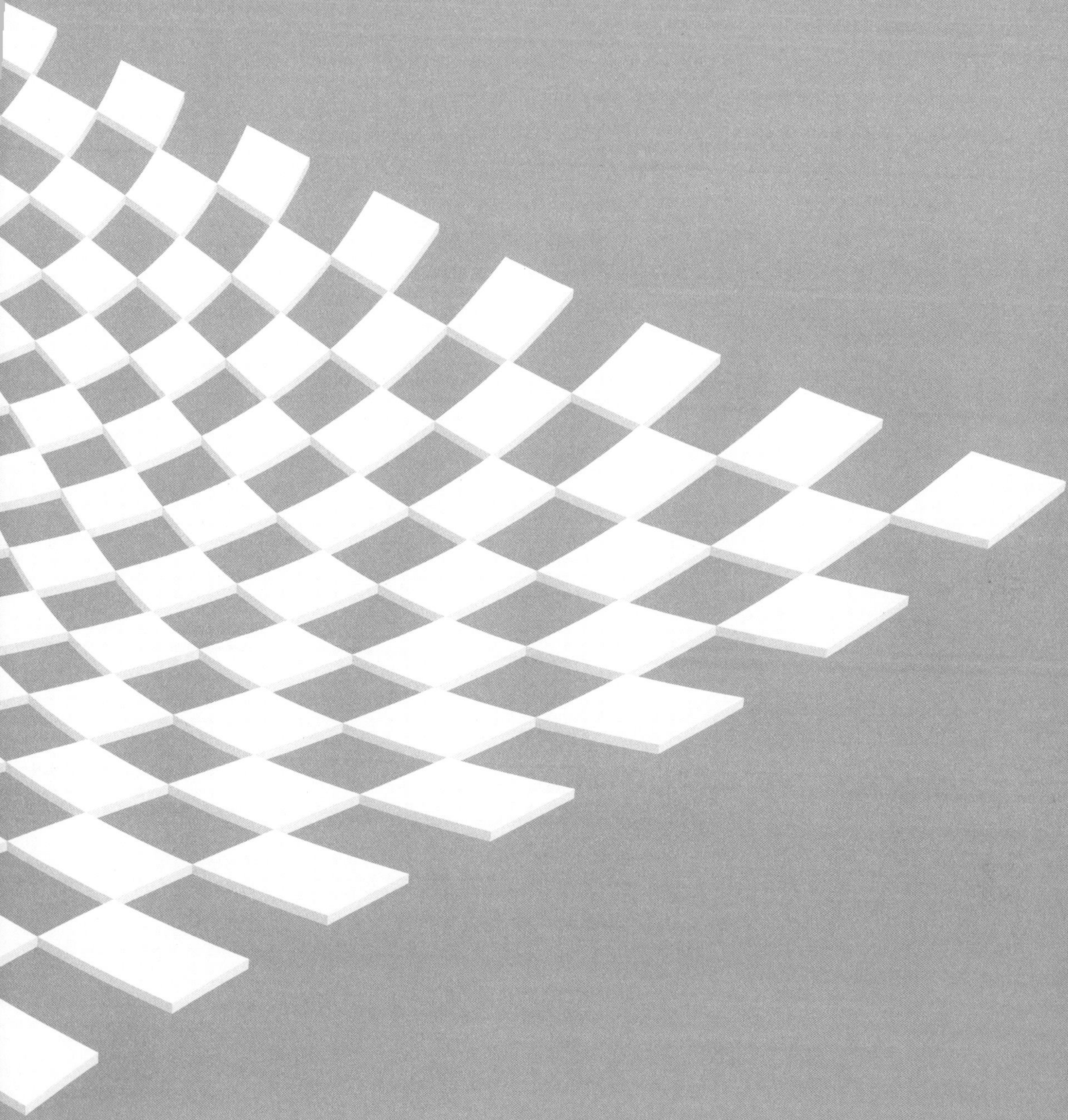

Hugh D. A. Goldring is a writer from Ottawa, Ontario, Algonquin territory. As one half of Petroglyph Studios, he works full time writing comics with social justice themes in partnership with scholars, unions, activists, and NGOs. He is part of the Ad Astra Comix publishing collective, which published his first graphic novel, *The Beast: Making a Living on a Dying Planet*. He was active in the Occupy movement and has been involved in several Food Not Bombs chapters. He has spent the last five years traveling across the United States, visiting with anti-fascists, migrant rights activists, and anti-capitalists, trying vainly to make sense of it all.

nicole marie burton is a comic artist and children's book illustrator living in Ottawa, Ontario. Her published works include *The Boy Who Walked Backwards*, *The Beast: Making a Living on a Dying Planet*, *Enemy Alien: A True Story of Life Behind Barbed Wire*, and *Coal Mountain*, part of the comics anthology *Drawn to Change: Graphic Histories of Working Class Struggle*. She is a founding member of the Ad Astra Comix publishing collective.

Dr. Erika Dyck is a professor and Canada Research Chair in the History of Health & Social Justice at the University of Saskatchewan. She is the author of *Psychedelic Psychiatry* (2008) and *Facing Eugenics* (2013), co-author of *Managing Madness* (2017) and *Challenging Choices* (2020), and co-editor of *Psychedelic Prophets* (2018) and *A Culture's Catalyst* (2016). She is also a member of the Chacruna Institute for Psychedelic Plant Medicines.